Computer-Aided Intelligent Diagnosis of Skin Melanoma

Shuli Guo · Xiaowei Song · Lina Han

# Computer-Aided Intelligent Diagnosis of Skin Melanoma

Springer

Shuli Guo
School of Automation
Beijing Institute of Technology
Beijing, China

Xiaowei Song
School of Mechatronic Engineering
North University of China
Taiyuan, China

Lina Han
Department of Cardiology
The Second Medical Center
Chinese PLA General Hospital
Beijing, China

ISBN 978-981-96-6134-3 ISBN 978-981-96-6135-0 (eBook)
https://doi.org/10.1007/978-981-96-6135-0



This Springer imprint is published by the registered company Springer Nature Singapore Pte Ltd.
The registered company address is: 152 Beach Road, #21-01/04 Gateway East, Singapore 189721, Singapore

*We heartily congratulate Academician of the Chinese Academy of Sciences, Prof. Huang Lin of Peking University for the 90th birthday.*

# Preface

Melanoma is responsible for approximately all 85% fatalities caused by skin cancer. During the initial stages of melanoma development, discernible symptoms are notably absent. The computer-aided intelligent modelling and diagnosis have a significant meaning for the skin melanoma. To address some interested issues on digital skin melanoma, such as color inaccuracies, structured noise disruption, and uneven feature point distribution in melanoma detection, some important techniques are proposed for interested region color correction, background hair removal, and image registration in the dermoscopic images. The ultimate aim is to enhance the precision of intelligent diagnosis of melanoma and related skin diseases.

Many important technologies are introduced as follows. Firstly, the multi-scale image gamma correction is proposed for the color correction of dermoscopic images. By employing smooth optimization and Lagrange duality, the above color correction problem is transformed into an unconstrained convex optimization problem, and the Newton iteration method is employed to solve the objective function and effectively converges towards an optimal solution. Secondly, a novel hair removal model, including the maximum variance fuzzy clustering and an improved Criminisi algorithm, is proposed for weak repair accuracy of hair extraction. The former is employed to separate the extracting regions from the surrounding similar ones, and the latter is enhanced by incorporating the characteristics of structural strength and data coherence. A color weighting sample block matching criterion is proposed to improve the prioritization of selected repair blocks. Thirdly, a total variation hair removal model is proposed for the structured noise within the skin lesion area, including the integrating texture spectrum iterative tensor voting and its optimization techniques. The above approaches, characterized by its manageable complexity, significantly enhance the accuracy of hair extraction. Finally, a novel dermoscopic image registration model is proposed for many registration issues, such as non-uniform visual field/angle, uneven feature point extraction, and weak image registration accuracy, including the adaptive SURF feature extraction and weighted kernel norm minimization fusion. It has been demonstrated that the proposed algorithm ensures accurate and seamless merging of the different images through extensive interferences and scene conditions.

This book will present more engineering models for digital medicine, which have the potential applications in the future. These models aim to make medicine sciences more AI and digital virtualization. This book will be a valuable guide for undergraduate students, graduate students, engineers and researchers in the fields of biomedical engineering, applied image processing and clinical medicine.

Beijing, China Shuli Guo

**Acknowledgements** We wish to thank those experts who have given us comments and discussion concerning these topics.

Special thanks go to the Academician of the Chinese Academy of Sciences, Prof. Huang Lin of Peking University, Academician of the Chinese Academy of Engineering, Prof. Chen Jie of Chinese Department of Education, Academician of the Chinese Academy of Engineering, Prof. Fu Mengyin of Nanjing University of Science and Technology, Prof. Irene Moroz from Oxford University, Prof. Si Ligeng of Inner Mongolia Normal University, Prof. Wang Long of Peking University, Prof. Ji Linhong of Tsinghua University, Prof. Yan Shaoze of Tsinghua University, Prof. Cao Xiankun of Education Department of Hainan Province, Prof. Ren Fujun of China Association for Science and Technology, Prof. Li Xiaoying, Prof. Liu Liang, Prof. Li Xingjie, Prof. Sheng Li, Prof. He Kunlun, Prof. Wang Chunxi, Prof. Luo Leiming of Chinese PLA General Hospital, and Prof. Ma Wanbiao of University of Science and Technology, Beijing. Prof. Wang Junzheng, Prof. Xia Yuanqing, Prof. Wang Zhaohua, Prof. Zhang Baihai, Prof. Sun Jian of Beijing Institute of Technology, Prof. Wei Yingbin of Hainan University, and Prof. Liu Zhonghe of Baotou Medical College.

We wish to thank our friends Prof. Chen Huiyang, Prof. Liu Mingpeng, Prof. He Jinxu, Prof. Fu Chuanyi of Hainan College of Software Technology, who have encouraged us to carry it out.

We wish to thank our graduate Ph.D. degree students Wang Hui, Wu Lei, Zhao Zhilei, Wu Yue, Cekderi Anil Baris, Jia Jiaoyu, Olentcevich Arina, Sheari Yashubu, Li Dongni and our master's degree graduate students Xue Jianing, Huang Haichun, Chao Yue, Huang Haitao.

We wish to thank Beijing Overseas Talents Program under the Grant J2024011, National Key Research and Development Program of China under the Grant 2017YFF0207400, Hainan Province Science and Technology Special Fund under the Grant ZDYF- 2021GXJS205, and Hainan College of Software Technology.

We also wish to take this opportunity to thank Dr. Huang Shuting of Dalian University of Technology, Dr. Hou Xinyu of Oxford University and Mrs. Tian Xin of Beijing University of Technology Affiliated High School for repeatedly reviewing the entire manuscript and giving their constructive comments.

We would like to acknowledge the support of Mr. Wayne Hu for taking care of the typing and preparation of this book's manuscript. Lastly, this book is dedicated to Viradasarani Natarajan and his colleagues for their active efforts.

Beijing, China
May 2024

Shuli Guo

**Competing Interests** The authors have no competing interests to declare that are relevant to the content of this manuscript.

# Introduction

During the initial stages of melanoma development, discernible symptoms are notably absent. Because the region with melanin deposition shares very similar characteristics with benign moles in terms of anatomical distribution, color and area, it is difficult to identify different skin diseases with naked eyes. The accuracy of intelligent diagnosis of melanoma is affected by the following interference information such as the low contrast between the lesion region and normal skin region, the unclear boundaries, the color deviations, the structured noise interference, the uneven distribution of feature points, small data sets, etc. In order to improve the melanoma recognition accuracy, some important novel models such as color correction, hair removal, image registration and classification recognition of dermoscopic images are proposed as follows.

Based on combination of gamma correction and multi-scale images, a color correction model is proposed to address color deviation in dermatoscopic images. Firstly, an objective function based on color deviation criterion is established, and the above model is transformed into an unconstrained convex optimization solution through the smoothing optimization and the Lagrangian duality. Secondly, Newton's iterative method is proposed to obtain the preliminary correction model of the image by solving the objective function; then, the obtained preliminary correction models are fused to achieve the expected color correction model. Finally, the experimental results demonstrate that the proposed model can realize the color correction while retaining the color features of the lesion region as much as possible. Furthermore, it is not sensitive to the setting of parameters, which ensures the stability and robustness of the dermatoscopic images.

Given deficiencies in the dermoscopic images such as the inaccurate extraction regions, the weak robustness and low repair accuracy, a hair removal model based on the maximum variance fuzzy clustering and the improved Criminisi algorithm is proposed. Firstly, the regional growth algorithm is proposed to address the discontinuity of the extraction region; secondly, the maximum variance fuzzy clustering is tried to solve excessively large extraction region when hair color is close to the surrounding area; Then the fuzzy membership function is designed to optimize the following problems such as the local optimum and weak robustness in hair clustering; and then the traditional Criminisi algorithm is combined with the structural strength and the data coherence characteristics, and color weight model is designed in matching sample blocks; finally, the ant colony algorithm is designed to optimize the search pathing during matching these blocks.

As the traditional hair extraction algorithms are susceptible to structured noise in the lesion region, a texture spectrum model is proposed based on the iterative tensor voting algorithm, which defines the attenuation function of the texture spectrum from the angle deviations between the voting machine and the receiver, so that the voting field scale is constantly updated during the iteration. It enables the feature points with the hair structure information to obtain more voting information and completely extract the hair structure of the dermatoscope. During hair repairing, the priori information of hair in the dermatoscope is first modeled. Then, an energy functional that satisfies the noise constraints is established, and the diffusion adjustment coefficients are designed to add to the regular term. And then, the Euler-Lagrange equation is used to solve the iterative model, and the adaptive parameters that affect the iterations are introduced, which can realize fast diffusing in the early iteration and slowing down in the late iteration. Finally, the experiments show the accuracy rate of the proposed hair extraction model is increased to 99.28% on average, which is better than other traditional algorithms. At the same time, its running time is less than other texture-based repair methods.

An image registration model based on adaptive SURF feature extraction and weighted kernel norm minimization fusion is proposed to overcome the multi-angle dermoscopic images registration. Firstly, the SURF algorithm is proposed to extract feature points from dermoscopic images, and the hunter prey optimization algorithm is used to adaptively evaluate the number of groups, layers, and Hessian determinant thresholds in the SURF algorithm. Secondly, the thin plate spline model is adapted for the coarse image registration, and at the same time, an improved random sampling consistency algorithm is used to remove pseudomatching points. And then, a weighted kernel norm fusion method is adopted to preserve the original color pixel information in the reference image and the image to be registered as much as possible, which can reduce the loss of the image and improve the visual effect of the fused image during the stitching process. Finally, the experiments show that the improved algorithms have good rotation invariance, scale invariance, and affine invariance features. The proposed algorithms can uniformly and stably extract feature points such as moles, scars, and hair. At the same time, they can apply to different interferences with good stability and robustness.

# Contents

# About the Authors

**Prof. Shuli Guo** was born in 1973 in Inner Mongolia, P.R. China. He received his bachelor degree (1995), master degree (1998) from Inner Mongolia Normal University and his Ph.D. degree from Peking University (2001) and worked as a postdoctoral researcher from January 2002 to April 2004 at Tsinghua University, as a researcher fellow from January 2008 to September 2008 at Akita Prefectural University, and as a postdoctoral researcher from September 2008 to September 2009 at Oxford University. His research interests include medical image/data analysis, typical chronic disease analysis, and remote health monitoring. And now he is the full professor of Beijing Institute of Technology, the head of China geriatric disease standardized diagnosis and treatment society of CAGG, the member of Chinese national technical committee for professional standardization. Recently, he has chaired seven Chinese national standards and five Chinese industry standards, more than 80 impactful papers, six monographs, 55 authorized Chinese patents, 23 authorized software copyrights. He obtained the second prize for Beijing Municipal Government, the third prize for military medical achievements, the third prize of science and technology of the Chinese Medical Association, and the third prize of Beijing Medical Science and Technology.

**Dr. Xiaowei Song** was born in 1993 in Shanxi Province, P.R. China. He received his Ph.D. degree from Beijing Institute of Technology (2024). And he is now working as a lecturer at North University of China. His research interests include medical image processing and modelling and telemedicine network standards. He has published about ten impactful paper, Chinese invention patents, software copyrights, and three Chinese national/industry standards.

**Prof. Lina Han** was born in 1973 in Jilin Province, P.R. China. She received her medicine bachelor degree (1995), medicine master degree (2000), and Ph.D. degree (2003) from Jilin University. She worked as a postdoctoral researcher from July 2003 to April 2005 at Chinese PLA General Hospital and as a research fellow from August 2008 to September 2009 at Kyoto University. And now, she works as a research fellow in Department of Cardiovascular Internal Medicine, the 2nd

Medicine Center of Chinese PLA General Hospital, and Chinese PLA Medical School. Her research interests focus on intelligent diagnosis of diseases and their medical solutions. Recently, she has published more than 100 impactful papers, seven monographs, 40 authorized Chinese patents, 15 authorized software copyrights, seven Chinese national standards and five Chinese industry standards. She obtained the first prize for Hainan Municipal Government, the second prize for Beijing Municipal Government, the first prize for military medical achievements, etc.

# Acronyms

| | |
|---|---|
| AC | Ant Colony Optimization Criminisi |
| AK | Actinic Keratosis |
| BCC | Basal Cell Carcinoma |
| BKL | Benign Keratosis |
| CO | Convolution Repair Algorithm |
| DF | Dermatofibroma |
| EO | Edge Operator |
| FC | Fuzzy Clustering |
| GCC | Gamma Correction with Constraints |
| GCMF | Gamma Correction, and Multi-scale Image Fusion |
| HPO | Hunter Prey Optimizer |
| IN | Linear Interpolation Algorithm |
| ISGC | Image Sharpening with Gamma Correction |
| MEL | Melanoma |
| MFC | Maximum Variance Fuzzy Clustering |
| MMCrCb | Mean of Medians of CrCb |
| MO | Morphological Operation |
| MT | Morphological Operation+Threshold Segmentation |
| NV | Nevus |
| PA | Pixel Accuracy |
| RANSAC | Random Sample Consensus |
| SCC | Squamous Cell Carcinoma |
| SIFT | Scale-Invariant Feature Transform |
| SOG | Shadow of Grey |
| TC | Traditional Criminisi algorithm |
| TV | Total Variation |
| VASC | Vascular Skin Disease |

# Chapter 1
# Image Processing Techniques for Skin Diseases

## 1.1 Skin Diseases and Dermatoscopy Images

As one of the largest organs of the human body, the skin itself occurs various types of skin diseases, and many other diseases that occur in human organs can also be characterized on the skin [1, 2]. At present, the incidence rate of skin diseases among Chinese people amounts to over 40%, which ranks the fourth among all diseases in terms of health and lifespan loss. Compared with other skin cancers with more higher incidence rates, such as basal cell carcinoma and squamous cell carcinoma, malignant melanoma is the most lethal disease among all skin diseases, whose incidence rate accounts for only 6.8–20% of all skin cancers, but spectacularly whose death rate reaches to about 85% due to skin cancer [3, 4].

Malignant melanoma is the most malignant tumor among all known skin diseases, and its essence is the malignant transformation of melanocytes, which can occur in any tissues or organs containing any melanocytes such as the skin, the mucosa, and mostly stems from the skin nevus. Due to the fact that the skin is the largest organ tissue in the anatomy and almost connects to all other organs, melanoma is highly prone to diffusing in the anatomy, with extremely poor healing effects, commonly known as the "king of cancer" [5]. For examples, there are over 100,000 melanoma cases per year in the United States of America with over 9000 deaths, over 13,000 melanoma cases per year in the Australia with approximately 1200 deaths and over 20,000 melanoma deaths per year in the European countries [6–8]. Although the incidence of melanoma in the China is relatively low, there are over 20,000 added cases per year. Therefore, global attention to melanoma should be strengthened [9].

Based on the characteristics of the relevant pathogenesis, origin, course, and prognosis of malignant melanoma, it can be divided into two categories: in situ malignant melanoma and invasive malignant melanoma [10]. The former is defined as tumor cells that are limited to the epithelial layer of the epidermis or mucosa, including malignant freckle like nevi, superficial diffuse in situ malignant melanoma, and limb in situ melanoma. The latter is defined as tumor cells that have broken through the

 
S. Guo et al., *Computer-Aided Intelligent Diagnosis of Skin Melanoma*,
https://doi.org/10.1007/978-981-96-6135-0_1

basal layer of the epidermis or mucosal epithelium, and infiltrated into the dermis and deeper layers, including superficial diffuse malignant melanoma, malignant freckle like melanoma, acromegaly melanoma, and nodular melanoma. In the early stages of malignant melanoma diseases such as in situ cancer, the survival rate can reach up to 98% through simple treatments such as surgical resection, while in the late stage, the survival rate decreases to less than 20% [11, 12], which greatly promotes the early-stage diagnosis techniques for skin diseases. However, the early symptoms of malignant melanoma are difficult to identify, which results to only an less than 60% accuracy rate for dermatologists performing unassisted visual examinations [13]. The dermatoscopy is the main tool for non-invasively detecting skin diseases, which can display the enlarged skin lesions and exhibit many advantages such as enlarged lesions details, deeper pathological layers, lower surface reflection rate, etc. Therefore, it has been the common skin diseases diagnostic technique, whose accuracy rate is significantly improved with compared to the unassisted examinations [14].

Since the dermatoscopy images clinical diagnose mainly depends on the subjective experiences of dermatologists and very poor reproducibility, the dermatologists are required to have rich clinical practice experiences, unless easily result to misdiagnosis or missed diagnosis [15]. Now there exist six common subjective diagnostic methods such as pattern analysis diagnostic method [16], ABCD criterion method [17], three-point feature diagnostic method [18], seven-point feature diagnostic method [19], Montessori diagnostic method [20], and CASH diagnostic rule [21]. Argenziano et al. [22] concludes that dermatologists with rich clinical diagnostic experiences reach to a 95% sensitivity and 75% specificity using the seven-point feature diagnosis method, while those with the limited diagnostic experiences do only 85% and 48%. The above sensitivity and specificity based on the ABCD criterion can reach to 85% and 66% respectively for experienced ones, while 95% and 27% for the inexperienced ones. The most effective pattern analysis method only reaches to the 76% accuracy rate for the experienced ones. It is well-known that the lower diagnostic rate further exacerbates the harm of melanoma in the world. Therefore, computer-aided melanoma modelling and diagnosis technologies based on dermatoscopy images [23, 24] can efficiently improve the diagnostic accuracy rate of skin tumors, which is very important and highly worth attempts.

## 1.2 Present Status and Challenges

At present, many scientists have focused on dermatoscopy image processing and intelligent recognition of melanoma, and achieved the following valuable progress.

### 1.2.1 Melanoma Image Processing and Intelligent Recognition

Melanoma mostly evolves from melanin nevi in the early stages, and even if detailed descriptions of the lesion area are obtained through dermatoscopy, the accurate recognition cannot be made. Different skin diseases can exhibit very similar characteristics in terms of anatomical distribution, color changes, and regional shapes [25, 26], which is characterized by asymmetric shapes, irregular edges, pigmentation, varying depths, over 6 mm diameters and so on. For example, Basal cell carcinoma exhibits slow growth and the highest occurrence frequency, which can occur in many regions such as the face and/or the neck, which is characterized by colored or coloring bumps of varying sizes, less than 10 mm diameter, and so on [27]. Squamous cell carcinoma often presents as papules, keratinized spots, or ulcers, which can evolve from advanced nodular or ulcerative tumors [28]. Photokeratosis is characterized as rough papules, about 10 mm-diameter plaques and irregular edges [29]. High similar visual features are difficult to classify with the naked eye, and even difficult to directly observe and diagnose for the dermatologists without the help of tools.

With the development of artificial intelligence (AI) technology, many excellent results have been achieved in the processing and distinguishing dermoscopic images using machine learning and deep learning. Huang et al. [30] developed a lightweight skin disease classification model that can be deployed on cloud platforms and mobile devices. The model's binary classification accuracy on the KCGMH dataset reached to 89.5%, its seven-classification accuracy on the HAM10000 dataset was 85.8%, and its five-classification accuracy on the KCGMH dataset was 72.1%.

Thunhofer et al. [31] developed a deep learning framework model for skin cancer detection using data augmentation techniques and five used neural network techniques, whose recognition rate on the HAM10000 dataset reached to 87.7%. Khan et al. [32] designed a 30- layer CNN model based on the HAM10000 dataset and proposed a new summation discriminant correlation analysis technique to fuse those features extracted from two fully connected layers. Then, an extreme learning machine classifier was used to classify the selected features, with an overall accuracy of 87.02%. Although deep learning has been extensively utilized in classifying dermatoscopic images, there are still many challenges that result in the low recognition rates, which limit its further application in the daily life. The main drawbacks with skin disease recognition based on dermatoscopy image include the low contrast ratio between the lesion regions and the normal regions, and the vague boundaries/edges, and simultaneously, the image is severely affected by interference information such as hair, which affects the image color deviation. And especially, there exit fewer cases/reports, which increases the difficulty of collecting dermatoscopic images and confines further exploration on skin cancers. Therefore, a series of dermatoscopic images processing techniques have been developed to improve the accuracy of skin disease classification using artificial diagnosis or deep learning techniques. Dermatoscopic image processing techniques generally include image denoising, color correction, image registration, and image segmentation.

When designing an intelligent diagnostic system for melanoma, the noises in dermatoscopic images mainly are derived from the hair interference, and removing the above noises caused by the hair is an important challenge. The contrast between the early lesion of melanoma and the normal skin regions is not very clear, such as blurred boundaries and regional hair occlusion, which exacerbate the challenge of extracting the lesion regions [33, 34]. For the melanoma recognition, hair removal is not the most critical link, but the hair impact on the color recognition, the texture recognition, and the boundary recognition of the lesion region cannot be ignored, so hair removal is an indispensable premise for skin lesion segmentation and recognition [29]. The color of dermatoscopic images is one of the most important features in skin diseases. Although the experienced dermatologists can to some extent eliminate the adverse effects of chromatic aberration, it poses serious challenges for designing the integrated intelligent recognition systems [35–37]. Due to chromatic aberration in skin color, dermatoscopy images exhibit significant differences from other medical images, for example, the same disease may exhibit different color deviations among different races, and even within the same race, or even across different ages and genders [38, 39]. In addition, the local skin temporary redness by the rupture of capillaries (i.e. the patient's frequently scratching the skin) does not belong to the color characteristics of the skin disease itself [40]. Therefore, it is necessary to correct the chromatic aberration of dermatoscopy images and eliminate or reduce it [41]. Similarly, due to the environmental dynamic changes such as the different positions or the poses of the photographed subjects, the lighting settings, and the different time periods, the captured images of the same skin region may vary [42, 43]. In order to compare the dermatoscopy mirror images taken at different times, it is necessary to register the images, locate the skin lesion regions, obtain complete skin lesion images, and achieve long-term skin lesion detection. Skin lesion segmentation refers to firstly extracting the skin lesion area from the dermatoscopy images, and then analyzing the lesion regions feature indicators to classify the dermatoscopy images and finally eliminating the interferences from other region features. At present, the segmentation techniques of the dermoscopic images mainly include threshold methods [44], region growing methods [45], deep learning methods [46], and others [47, 48]. Among them, deep learning networks represented by the U-Nets and their improved networks have been widely exploited in the dermoscopic images segmentation, and their combinations with other classification networks greatly improve the recognition rate of the melanoma.

Among these dermoscopic image processing algorithms, the image segmentation is relatively mature and can meet the general requirements for extracting lesion regions in most scenarios. Until now, it takes storage of color correction, hair extraction & repair, and image registration for dermatoscopy images as research objects.

Therefore, for the computer-aided melanoma modelling and diagnosis technology based on the dermatoscopy images, many important issues, such as color correction, hair extraction and repair, image registration, and classification recognition will be conducted. The development of the mentioned four related items is listed below.

### 1.2.2 Color Correction on Dermatoscopy Images

The basic principle of dermatoscopy is to observe the relevant characteristics of skin tissues through the magnifying glass [27, 49]. When using dermatoscopes in different environments, due to the influence of different environments such as the sunshine temperature deviations, the light angle, the photography parameters, the refraction and /or the reflection under different polarizations of artificial light sources, there exist significant deviations in the dermatoscope images for the same patient [35–37].

The color correction is to remove the influence of interference factors to obtain the true color characteristics of the observed object, which is also known as the color constancy calculation [50].

The Retinex color constancy theory proposed by Land E. H. [51–53] is one of the most fundamental theories. He considers that the object's color is only determined by its inherent surface color characteristics, that is the light reflection coefficient on the object surface and is independent of the human eye. The Color constancy is a physiological characteristic possessed by the human eye, which can infer the true color of objects from the external conditions. However, the related image acquisition devices do not have the adjustment function and easily causes the color deviation in the obtained images. Therefore, it is necessary to eliminate the influence of color deviations in the lighting condition for the color correction. The Lambert reflection model is one of the main tools for the unsupervised color constancy based on the related color underlying images features [54], which can be used to estimate the illumination chromaticity of images. For the vast majority of unsupervised color constancy algorithms, it is currently required to set the corresponding constraints to ensure that the objective function can obtain a definite solution. The white patch algorithm [55] assumes that the maximum value of the color channel is directly related to the brightest region of the image. The grey world theory [56] assumes that the average values of the three color channels in the RGB images with rich color changes are basically equal. The premise of the grey world method is to assume that the average light reflection by the physical objects in nature is generally gray. The color balance algorithm can eliminate the effect of ambient light from the image and obtain the ideal target image during processing the images. These above theories together basically form the color constancy algorithm [57–59].

Due to the boundedness of the above theory in the practice, Finlayson et al. [60] further proposed the shadow of grey algorithm, which mainly set the white patch algorithm and the grey world algorithm into the same frame through adjusting the Minkowski norms, whose essence is that the weight assigned to image pixels is positively correlated with the pixel values of the image.

Gijsenij et al. [61] proposed the Grey Edge algorithm, which assumes that the mean surface reflectance of objects in the scene presents no color deviations, thus unifying the Gray World, the White Patch, and the Shade of Grey into a Grey Edge model. Once the possible scenes meet the above assumptions, many ideal results can be achieved. However, there is a significant deviation between the actual situation and the above assumptions for skin mirror color correction. Especially, there exist the consequence that affects the subjective quality of the image, such as the decreased saturation and the low brightness after color correcting.

On the basis of the above algorithms, many color correction optimized methods have been proposed. For example, Forsyth et al. [62] proposed the gamut mapping algorithm and its improved algorithm [63] falling within supervised color constancy algorithms, which assumed that the possible color range on the object surface under a given light source was bounded. Brainard et al. [64] proposed the color constancy calculation based on Bayesian theory by estimating the probability model of the surface reflectance distribution of objects on the scene. Rizzi et al. [65] proposed the automatic color equalization algorithm, which utilized the computational model of the human visual system. This method not only integrated the grayscale world and the global balance mechanism of white patches, but also achieved local filtering effects by considering the color space distribution in the image. It easily adapted to large-scale lighting varying conditions, effectively extracted visual information from the surrounding environments, and more important, achieved good experimental results in various color correction tasks. Babbar et al. [66] proposed a color correction model based on alternating the least squares and the root polynomials to reduce errors among the references and the target images, improved the image quality, and increased the realism of images.

The above algorithms are only designed for color correction algorithms in a single scene. However, there are generally multiple color deviations among images, and the single-type assumptions and/or constraints in color correction algorithms are difficult to meet practical correction needs. In order to combine the advantages of different algorithms and meet different needs as much as possible, an image fusion method is proposed to blend the obtained different correction images [67–70]. Zhang et al. [67] proposed an underwater image enhancement fusion method based on the Retinex color correction and the details preservation technology. Ma et al. [71] proposed a different color spaces fusion method based on CLAH, which mainly enhanced the original image to be processed by using the contrast limited adaptive histogram equalization and the Sobel edge detector in the YIQ and HIS color spaces, respectively, and then fused the two processed images together to obtain the final image. Ghani et al. [69] proposed homomorphic filtering and recursive overlap methods to adjust the brightness of the image and stretch the overlapping blocks of the image channel, respectively. Finally, they fused the processed images and obtained good results. Cheng et al. [70] fused the four color constancy algorithms and obtained good estimation results.

With the development of artificial intelligence, deep learning has made significant progresses in image color correction. Compared with the traditional enhancement algorithms, deep learning does not require some assumptions on the images, and the trained network can directly perform color correction on the image without the need of additional tuning. Wu et al. [72] proposed a novel structure decomposition network for color correction and enhancement of underwater images, using preliminary enhancement networks including high-frequency enhancement networks, low-frequency enhancement networks, as well as fine-grained networks to optimize the color of underwater images. Jiang et al. [73] proposed an efficient unsupervised generative adversarial network model, which utilized a series of methods such as the global/local discriminator structure, the self-regularization perceptual loss fusion, and the attention mechanism to solve the aporia of weak light image enhancement. The non-paired training process was regularized by inputting information extracted from the image itself. Liu et al. [74] proposed a generative adversarial network model for image color correction processing, which extracted multi-scale features of the image and then enhanced local features of each scale with the global features, thereby improved the network's performances in color correction and detail preservation. For the image color correction, the vast majority of deep learning adopted the generative adversarial networks, because they were easily compatible with different network structures and efficiently learned features of the obtained samples [75, 76]. However, Training the generative adversarial networks is complex and unstable, which requires a large number of datasets. And simultaneously, it is well-known that the different images often require different lighting conditions and color spaces, which makes it difficult for the deep learning models accurately to normalize images. The existed models greatly confine the application of deep learning in the color correction.

For the skin color correction, it is difficult to compile the standard images to form a complete training dataset, so machine learning algorithms are more widely used in this field. Shirai et al. [77] proposed an automatic image correction method for the portrait photos, which improved the consistency of facial skin color by restraining skin color changes caused by the background color. Berbar et al. [78] proposed the MMCrCb (Mean of Medians of CrCb) to address the issue of skin color deviations after the facial images exposure to illumination reflection. Compared to the underwater image color correction, the color deviations in the dermatoscopic images was not yet sufficiently addressed [79–81]. Many urgent and important issues need to solve, such as image color deviations, or color differences caused by light intensity, the equipment parameters or the color rendering equipment, as well as significant differences of the skin disease base-colors among different populations caused by the differences in skin color, the lesions, and the individual differences.

### *1.2.3 Hair Recognition and Repair in Melanoma*

The basic method for identifying melanoma was the ABCDE criterion [19, 82]. The presence of hair mainly leaded to some changes of the extracted lesion regions, including asymmetry of the lesion regions, irregularity of the lesion edges, uneven color of the lesion regions (i.e. hair darkened the color of the hair regions), and significant enlargements of the extracted lesion regions. The above results greatly reduced the success rate of melanoma recognition [7, 83].

The traditional hair removal algorithm in the dermoscopic images mainly consists of two steps. The first step is to detect and remove hair pixels in the image, and the second step is to repair the removed hair pixel information. The main methods for detecting hair include median filtering [84], morphological operations [85], and edge detection based algorithms such as using Canny operators [86], Prewitt operators

[87], and Stinger line detection [88] to detect interference noise signals such as hair. Traditional hair removal algorithms include median filtering [84], morphological operations [89], bilinear interpolation [90], and neighborhood pixel replacement [87]. The above several algorithms, such as median filtering and morphological operation, can be used in hair detection and repair, but simultaneously also cause some defects such as image blurring and color anomalies. Although these above basic methods can to some extent remove the impact of hair, their repair effects are very poor, and even bring negative benefits when the hair texture is more complex.

Abbas et al. [91] used Gaussian derivatives to detect hair regions in the CIELab color space, applied morphological operations to connect missing hair regions, eliminated small and circular holes, and filled gaps between lines. And simultaneously they used some methods based on the coherence transport for hair restoration.

Huang et al. [92] applied a multi-scale curve matching filter for denoise, used a lagged threshold method to detect hair regions, and applied the region growth and the linear discriminant analysis to recover missing information after removing hair through combining the pixel color information in the CIELab color space.

Biblioni et al. [93] used an adaptive histogram equalization algorithm to improve the contrast of image brightness, and then used a soft color morphology operator to detect hair in the CIELab color space. During the repair phase, the missing pixels were restored based on the arithmetic mean of the modified open/closed morphology transformation.

In order to further improve the accuracy of hair removal algorithms, Satheesha et al. [94] detected hair using a quadratic curve. Koehoorn et al. [95] proposed a multi-level threshold method, which used gap detection algorithms to locate hair for each threshold, and then combined all results to determine a single mask. Mirzaalian et al. [96] applied the Markov random field theory and multi-label optimization for hair feature extraction and image enhancement. Mahmood et al. [97] only used a Canny edge detector to generate binary masks for hair in the red channel, and then used the Polygons Impainting method to complete hair restoration. Das et al. [98] processed images at both grayscale and RGB scales. Based on the edge detection characteristics, circular masks were generated to remove artifacts. The images were then repaired using normalization techniques. Finally, the hair repair was completed by calculating the minimum distance between adjacent pixels based on the frequency of pixel appearance in the RGB image.

Despite the wide variety of existed algorithms, the hair removal has not yet been perfectly solved. For hair extraction, the existed algorithms still face the following issues such as the inability to adaptively extract hair regions, hair extraction intervals, and the extraction of fake hair.

Medioni et al. [99] proposed the tensor voting method, which can extract many interest region complex interference information such as intersections, curves, and surfaces through structural restructuring without relying on a specific model [100]. Although the tensor voting algorithms could directly obtain the images curve structure in many cases, when the image contrast was too low or the interference is too large, it could not be fully extracted through a single vote and needs to be revoted until the complete curve structure information was obtained [101, 102]. Loss et al.

[103] combined tensor voting and iterative voting together for the uncertain curve structure of medical cell membranes and obtained the good experimental results. Compared to other images, dermoscopic images have more complex texture structures and lower contrasts, and the tensor voting algorithms cannot directly be applied to hair detection, and further be required to improve.

The existed algorithms are unable to repair the texture details of dermoscopic images, which will destroy the edge features of the lesion regions and thus have a certain adverse impact on the melanoma recognition. The image restoration algorithms based on textures or structural information are the most widely utilized. For example, the Criminisi algorithm, as one of the most classical texture restoration methods, replaced the damaged regions with the searched sample blocks according to a certain order [104, 105]. In practice, the Criminisi algorithm requires complex computational processing in both priority and best matching template search, and easily results in a lengthy calculation process. Xu et al. [106] used the sparse linear combination to represent the current block to be repaired, and reduced the required time. Hesabi et al. [107] improved the original algorithm by modifying the priority and adding the feature information such as gradient and divergence when calculating inter block distances. Criminisi et al. [108] proposed an optimal priority algorithm, in which the confidence of the pixel values to be repaired was updated through a similar repair information propagation method, and the actual pixel values were calculated through sample block synthesis. Jin et al. [109] proposed a patch sparsity image restoration that achieved better performances in restoring missing structures of the images. Although the Criminisi algorithm has a relatively complete theoretical system, there are still a series of challenges that need to be solved in specific application fields.

The image structure restoration algorithm mainly utilizes the partial differential equations for image restoration algorithms, such as the BSCB restoration algorithm [110], the TV restoration algorithm [111, 112], the CDD restoration algorithm [113], etc. This type of algorithm diffuses the structure of undamaged areas to the damaged ones by calculating the characteristics of the damaged ones. For the image restoration problems, the basic approach is to use non-local regularized quadratic functions and non-local total variational functions to establish non-local regularized models between many image blocks in the following literatures. Lanza et al. [42] studied a class of variational model image restoration inverse problems, which assumed that the additive noise model and the image gradient amplitude followed a generalized normal distribution, and the probability density function was flexibly characterized by two parameters. Liang et al. [114] designed a non-convex sparse optimization model based on the proximal alternating direction multiplier method, and performed $L_0$ sparse regularization on the binary masks, where the total variation term was used to describe the clean image at the bottom layer, and the fidelity term L2 regularization was used to solve the given blind coating problem. Although the above algorithms have improved its adaptability by improving the energy functional based on the total variation method, there are still some problems such as a high number of repair iterations and the required long time.

### 1.2.4 Current Status of Image Registration in Skin Melanoma

Melanoma monitoring is a long-term process that requires collecting skin lesion images and location distribution at different time periods to monitor changes in the appearance and distribution of lesions. Due to the changing conditions during each acquisition process, the images of the same skin regions collected at different times will inevitably be different. The purpose of image registration is to solve the geometric transformation relationship between two or among more images containing the overlapping part [115, 116]. The traditional image registration algorithms are designed based on grayscale characteristics, frequency domains and/or features.

The image grayscale registration algorithm is to analyze the grayscale distribution information between the images, and to construct their similarity measurement indicators based on the grayscale distribution information, and to achieve the maximum or the minimum similarity indicators by optimizing the transformation parameters. According to different similarity measurement indicators, the image grayscale registration algorithms can be divided into the absolute mean deviations algorithm [117], the absolute accumulation algorithm [118], the error accumulation of squares algorithm [119], the mean error accumulation of squares algorithm [120], the normalized product correlation algorithm [121], and the sequential similarity detection methods [122]. In terms of maximizing or minimizing the similarity metrics, there are many image grayscale registration optimization algorithms. For example, Gong et al. [123] used the Marquardt Levenberg search strategy to solve the registration parameters, Gharbia et al. [124] used the particle swarm optimization algorithm to complete image registration, and Chen et al. [125] proposed a medium/ low resolution remote sensing image registration algorithm based on the quantum particle swarm optimization and the robust mutual information region.

By combining different similarity metrics and different optimization algorithms, different image registration algorithms can be constructed. There are two key factors that can affect the performance of the algorithms such as the accuracy of similarity measurement indicators, and the optimization efficiency of related optimization algorithms. The main challenges faced by these algorithms are how to select appropriate similarity measurement indicators and related optimization algorithms based on the specific usage scenarios.

The basic principle of the image frequency domain registration was to convert the image into a frequency domain representation [68, 126], and then performed the image registration operations in the frequency domain. Huang et al. [127] utilized the images edge features and the fast Fourier transform registration algorithms to obtain fast coarse registration, and then combined the enhanced correlation coefficient registration algorithm with the segmentation definition to register the obtained coarse registration results, and finally achieved the accurate registration. Through combining accelerated robust feature algorithms with logarithmic polarity phase correlation methods, Qu [128] proposed a new method that utilized a two-step iterative phase correlation algorithm for local region extraction and reuse, avoiding excessive computation and redundant requirements for image features, and effectively improving the accuracy of registration. Combining the image spectrum with a regular grid, Yu et al. [129] proposed the scale invariant feature transform (SIFT), an image registration method, which was used to extract a large number of feature points in high-frequency regions of the image, and a fine spatial distribution of regular grid features to ensure the distribution of feature points uniform. Their global correspondence error checking was used to remove incorrect matching pairs, and the image registration frequency-domain method had good performances for large-scale image translation, rotation, and scaling operations. However, the image registration frequency-domain algorithm is not prefect for processing large deformations or non-rigid transformations, which greatly limits the application of the above algorithms.

Currently, feature registration algorithms are the most widely used image registration algorithms. Its process includes extracting features that can clearly reflect the image characteristics, calculating the similarity between the extracted features, completing image feature matching based on the obtained similarity, and obtaining the transformation parameters of the image.

The commonly used features that reflect image characteristics include point features [129] (such as region corners, line intersections, image inflection points, etc.), line features [130] (such as skin lesion boundaries, hair, etc.), and region features [131] (such as faces, skin lesion areas, etc.). For specific applications, different features can be selected based on different types of images. Among them, surfaces and line features are more complex in the extraction process, with complex algorithms, poor stability, and poor robustness. Therefore, point features become the most commonly used features. Feature registration requires feature extraction, feature description, and feature matching operations.

Feature point extraction generally involves extracting corners of the image, intersections of lines, centroids of regions, inflection points of curves, and local extremum points. Common image feature point extraction algorithms include BRIEF operator [102], SUSAN operator [132], FREAK operator [133], BRISK operator [134], ORB operator [135], etc. They are mainly used for image edge detection and corner detection in the fields of image processing and computer vision. When describing feature points, the SIFT algorithm has become a well-known and effective algorithm due to its good scale invariance, rotation invariance, and robustness. A large number of improved post algorithms have been proposed based on this framework.

Zhang [136] used the weighted mean ratio operator to calculate uniform gradient information, and then extracted image feature points. Ordóñez [137] used the maximum stable extremum region feature detection algorithm to partition the image, and effectively utilized the information contained in different spectral bands to enhance image registration, and ultimately achieved image registration combining with the original SIFT. Based on structural tensors for the image registration, Divya [138] proposed a SIFT algorithm that constructed a scale layer using tensor diffusion technology. Although the SIFT algorithm has wide advantages, it requires a large number of feature descriptor comparisons during the feature matching stage, which results in the high computational complexity. The SURF algorithm mainly accelerates the process of feature point detection and descriptor computation by using the integrated images and the fast Hessian matrix detection methods, which greatly reduces the computational complexity of the SIFT algorithm, and improves its computational speed.

Feature point matching first calculates the distance or similarity among feature points in the registered image, then selects the closest feature point as the matching point, and removes incorrect registration points through the model's matching degree to ultimately complete image registration. The commonly used metrics for evaluating the similarity between feature points currently include the Euclidean distance, the Minkowski distance, and the spectral angular distance, where the Euclidean distance [139] and the spectral angular distance [140] represent the absolute distance and cosine value of the angle between the two vectors, respectively. The feature point registration algorithm is required to meet the consistency of the determined rules, which can remove those incorrect matched points based on the given rules.

The most representative work is the Random Sample Consensus (RANSAC) algorithm. This algorithm fits the model by randomly selecting a subset of data, and estimates the correct registration point based on the consistency between the fitted model and the data by statistically analyzing the sample points to meet the consistency criteria. Those algorithms such as maximum likelihood estimation sampling consistency [141] are improved by adding some constraints to the RANSAC. The traditional RANSAC algorithm relies on the number of iterations and the set threshold to keep the model accuracy. Due to the limitation of iteration times, the RANSAC algorithm can only obtain the optimal solution under the set iteration number, that is, the confidence of the result is positively correlated with the iteration number. When the data contains a large number of noise points or the model requires high accuracy, the number of iterations will exponentially increase, which will lead to the model spending more time. If the number of iterations is too small, it will lead to the end of the iteration before finding the optimal result, and even result in the incorrect fitting solutions.

## 1.3 Scientific Issues and Challenges

### *1.3.1 Scientific Issues*

In the early stages of melanoma, there are no obvious symptoms. For example, the melanin deposition region has very similar characteristics with the benign nevi, and different skin diseases can present very similar characteristics in anatomical distribution, color, and area, making it difficult to classify with the naked eye. For the dermatoscopy images, the contrast between the lesion region and the normal is low, and the edges are unclear. The classification can also easily be affected by interference information such as hair and abnormal image colors. The melanoma faces the following scientific issues:

Due to the variations in daytime color temperature, light angles, photography parameters, as well as the refraction and reflection interference of artificial light sources under different polarizations, there are many color deviations in the dermatoscope images. The construction or the solution of color correction objective functions, as well as the fusion between detailed texture features and basic color brightness information in the multi-scale images, are the key scientific issues in solving color interference.

The presence of hair can cause asymmetric shapes, irregular edges, uneven color, and enlarged lesion areas in the extracted lesion region. Therefore, it is necessary to remove hair from skin mirror images to ensure the accuracy of skin disease detection. The threshold or morphological operation extraction algorithms in hair removal mainly suffer from the challenges of over segmentation and under segmentation. In practice, the Criminisi algorithm faces the issues such as priority and fitness of skin mirror images when searching for the optimal matching template.

Due to low contrast and structured noises between hair and skin lesion regions, inter class variance fuzzy clustering cannot solve many challenges such as extraction obstruction and long running time. The tensor voting algorithm to extract hair structure mainly faces adaptive difficulties such as the inability to obtain complete structural information and the size of the voting domain through one voting iteration. The total variation algorithm for hair repair also faces how to use the diffusion coefficients in adjusting the iteration speed of the algorithm.

When using the SURF algorithm for the image registration, how to select parameters such as the Hessian matrix determinant thresholds for extracting an appropriate number of feature points is involved. For the traditional feature point matching algorithms, the model accuracy relies on the iteration times and the set thresholds, and how to balance iteration times and the confidence is another hot for the image registration.

### *1.3.2 Main Research Frame*

In response to the above issues, many interested efforts are conducted on color correction, hair removal, and image registration of dermatoscopy images, whose overall frame is as follows:

In Chap. 2, a color correction model based on gamma correction and multi-scale image fusion is proposed. Firstly, using the color deviation as the objective function for gamma correction, the constrained objective function is transformed into an unconstrained convex optimization problem through the smooth optimization of the objective function, the Lagrangian duality and so on; Then, the objective function is solved using the Newton iteration method, and the initial value dependency problem in the Newton iteration method is solved through using the binary method to obtain the preliminary correction results of the image; Finally, the preliminary corrected images are fused to obtain the color correction of dermoscopic image.

In Chap. 3, a dermoscopic image hair removal models based on the maximum inter class variance fuzzy clustering and the improved Criminisi algorithm are proposed.

Firstly, the region growth algorithm is used to solve the extracted region discontinuities; Secondly, the maximum inter class variance fuzzy clustering method is used to solve the excessively large extraction regions when the color of hair is close to the surrounding area; Fuzzy membership functions are used to solve problems such as easily falling into local optima and poor robustness of hair extraction for the clustering optimization; Then, the priority of the traditional Criminisi algorithm is fused with the structural strength and the data coherence, and color weights are standardized in matching the sample blocks; Finally, the ant colony algorithm is designed to optimize the search path in matching blocks.

In Chap. 4, the dermoscopic image hair removal models based on the texture spectrum iterative tensor voting and the optimized total variation algorithm are proposed. By combining the texture spectrum of the image and redefining the attenuation function in the tensor voting algorithm, the more voting information on the points can be obtained on the hair structure in the image during the iteration process, and further infer more accurate hair structure information. In the process of hair repair, the prior information of hair noises are firstly modeled in the dermatoscopy images; An energy functional is established that satisfies the noise constraint conditions, and the diffusion adjustment coefficient is defined in the regularization term; An iterative formula is obtained through the Euler–Lagrange equation with defining the adaptive parameters that vary with the number of iterations, and finally the improved image restoration speed and/or quality is achieved.

In Chap. 5, a dermoscopic image registration model combining the adaptive SURF feature extraction with the weighted kernel norm minimization fusion is proposed. Firstly, the SURF algorithm is used to extract feature points from dermoscopic images, and the hunter-prey optimization algorithm is used to adaptively calculate the number of groups, layers, and Hessian determinant thresholds in the SURF algorithm improves the stability and robustness of feature point extraction; The thin plate spline model method is used to image coarse registration, and an improved random sampling consistency algorithm is used to remove pseudo matching points from the feature point set of the obtained coarse registration, which improve the accuracy and efficiency of image registration; The weighted kernel norm fusion method is used, and the original color pixel information in the reference image and the image to be registered are preserved as much as possible, which reduce the loss of the image during the stitching process and strength the visual effect of the fused image.

## References

1. Li X, Liu C, He C. Clinical diagnosis and treatment of skin and sexually transmitted diseases. Wuhan: Hubei Science and Technology Press; 2023.
2. Ye X, Zhu H, Wang J. Diagnosis and treatment standards for common skin diseases. Guangzhou: Sun Yat sen University Press; 2023.
3. Fan D. Chinese Integrated Diagnosis and Treatment Guidelines for Cancer (CACA) in 2022, melanoma. Tianjin: Tianjin Science and Technology Press; 2022.

4. Han H, Gade A, Ceci FM, et al. Superfinancial radiation therapy for non-metalloma skin cancer: a review. Dermatol Rev. 2022;3(6):409–17.
5. Marks R, Motley R. Common Skin Diseases 18th edition. CRC Press, 2019
6. Richard M, Paul C, Nijsten T, et al. Prevalence of most common skin diseases in Europe: a population based study. Journal of the European Academy of Dermatology Vennerology. 2022;36(7):1088–96.
7. Cariti C, Merli M, Avallone G, et al. Melanoma management during the COVID-19 pandemic: a literature review and single center experience. Cancers. 2021;13(23):6071.
8. Yang DD, Borsky K, Jani C, et al. Trends in keratinocyte skin cancer incidence, morality, and burden of disease in 33 countries between 1990 and 2017. Br J Dermatol. 2023;188(2):237–46.
9. Monday Y, Mengyuan W, Weicheng Y, et al. Interpretation of 2022 US Cancer Statistics Report and Comparison of Cancer Epidemic in China and the United States. Electronic Journal of Comprehensive Tumor Therapy. 2022;8(2):54–63.
10. Castellon MJ. Pocket Guide to Malignant Melanoma. Plastic Reconstructive Surgery. 2003;112(5):1479.
11. Qi Z, Si L. New progress in the treatment of malignant melanoma. Chin Clin Oncol. 2019;46(5):213–7.
12. Miller K D, Nogueira L, Mariotto A B, et al. Cancer treatment and survival statistics, 2019. CA: a cancer journal for clinicians, 2019, 69 (5): 363–385
13. Takidin A, Schneider J, Yang Y, et al. Artistic intelligence for skin cancer detection: scoring review. J Med Internet Res. 2021;23(11):1438–8871.
14. Johr RH, Stolz W. Diagnostic Essentials and Illustrations of Dermatoscopy. Shanghai: Shanghai Science and Technology Press; 2023.
15. Ahmad N, Shah JH, Khan MA, et al. A novel framework of multiclass skin region recognition from dermoscopic images using deep learning and interpretable AI. Front Oncol. 2023;13:11151257.
16. Ramji R, Oakley A, Rademaker M. Morphological evolution in melanoma in situ using revised pattern analysis. Pigment Cell Melanoma Research. 2021;34(2):163–73.
17. Chatterjee S, Dey D, Munshi S, et al. Dermatological expert system implementing the ABCD rule of dermoscopy for skin disease identification. Expert Syst Appl. 2021;167: 114204.
18. Ludzik J, Becker AL, Lee C, et al. Augmenting segmented region assessment results with the three point dermoscopy checklist to improve segmented region triage. Skin Research Technology. 2022;28(6):877.
19. Congdon NM, Davis CM. A systematic review of the frequency of features of the seven point checklist in protected culinary medicine: The importance of change. Skin Health and Disease. 2023;3(6):295.
20. Menzies SW. A method for the diagnosis of primary cancer using surface microscopy. Dermatological clinics. 2001;19(2):299–305.
21. Di Meo N, Stinco G, Bonin S, et al. CASH algorithm verse 3-point checklist and its modified version in evaluation of melanocytic segmented skin sections: the 4-point checklist. J Dermatol. 2016;43(6):682–5.
22. Argenziano G, Soyer HP, Chimenti S, et al. Dermoscopy of segmented skin sections: results of a consensus meeting via the Internet. J Am Acad Dermatol. 2003;48(5):679–93.
23. Pham T-C, Luong C-M, Hoang V-D, et al. AI performed every mathematician in dermatological diagnosis, using an optimized deep CNN architecture with custom mini batch logic and loss function. Sci Rep. 2021;11(1):17485.
24. Yu Z, Nguyen J, Nguyen TD, et al. Early melanoma diagnosis with sequential dermoscopic images. Signal Processing Laboratory, Swiss Federal Institute of Technology, Lausanne. 2021;41(3):633–46.
25. Fontanillas P, Alipanahi B, Furlotte NA, et al. Disease risk scores for skin cancer. Nat Commun. 2021;12(1):160.
26. Cives M, Manavola F, Lospaluti L, et al. Non melanoma skin cancers: Biological and clinical features. Int J Mol Sci. 2020;21(15):5394.

27. Lee DJ, Faries MB. Practical manual for dermal and surgical management. Switzerland: Springer; 2021.
28. Warszawik Hendzel O, Olszewska M, Maj M, et al. Non invasive diagnostic techniques in the diagnosis of square cell cancer. Journal of Dermatological Case Reports. 2015;9(4):89.
29. Travers JB, Poon C, Rohrbach DJ, et al. Non volatile mosaic imaging of active skin damage using spatial frequency domain imaging. Biomed Opt Express. 2017;8(6):3045–52.
30. Huang H, Hsu BWY, Lee CH, et al. Development of a light weight deep learning model for cloud applications and remote diagnosis of skin cancer. J Dermatol. 2021;48(3):310–6.
31. Thunhofer Hemsi K. Dom í nguez E. A Convolutional Neural Network Framework for Accurate Skin Cancer Detection Neural Processing Letters. 2021;53(5):3073–93.
32. Khan M A, Muhammad K, Sharif M I, et al. Intelligent fusion associated skin region localization and classification for smart healthcare. Neural Computing and Applications, 2021: 1–16
33. Pereira AR, Collgros H, Guitera P, et al. Melanomas of the scale: is hair coverage preventing early diagnosis? Int J Dermatol. 2021;60(3):340–6.
34. Sardana K, Chakravarty P, Goel K. Optimal management of common acquired melanocytic nevi (moles): current perspectives. Clinical, Cosmetic and Investigational Dermatology, 2014: 89–103
35. Munjal A, Ferguson N. Skin Cancer in Skin of Color. Dermatological Clinics. 2023;41(3):481–9.
36. Sreelatiha T, Subramanyam M, Prasad MG. Shape and color feature based melanoma diagnosis using dermoscopic images. J Ambient Intell Humaniz Comput. 2021;12:5371–80.
37. Pritscher CP. Skin Color. Bioengineering of the Skin: CRC Press; 2020. p. 29–40.
38. Gutierrez D, Gaulding JV, Motta Beltran A, et al. Photodermatoses in skin of color. Journal of the European Academy of Dermatology and Vennerology. 2018;32(11):1879–86.
39. Lallas A, Reggiani C, Argenziano G, et al. Dermoscopic nevus patterns in skin of color: a prospective, cross sectional, morphological study in individuals with skin type V and VI. Journal of the European Academy of Dermatology and Vennerology. 2014;28(11):1469–74.
40. Ezenwa E, Stein JA, Krueger L. Dermoscopic features of neoplasms in skin of color: A review. International Journal of Women's Dermatology. 2021;7(2):145–51.
41. Razmjoy N, Razmjoy S, Vahedi Z, et al. Skin color segmentation based on artificial neural network improved by a modified grasshopper optimization algorithm. Methodology and Optimization in Computer and Electrical Engineering, 2021: 169–185
42. Lanza A, Pragliola M, Sgallari F. Automatic fidelity and regulation terms selection in variant image restoration. BIT Numerical Mathematics, 2021: 1–34
43. Xu X, Geng S. Blind Image Painting with Mixture Noise Using $\ell$ 0 and Total Regulation. Computational and Mathematical Methods in Medicine, 2022: 3180612
44. Ganster H, Pinz P, Rohrer R, et al. Automated melanoma recognition. Signal Processing Laboratory, Swiss Federal Institute of Technology, Lausanne. 2001;20(3):233–9.
45. Wong A, Scharcanski J, Fieguth P. Automatic Skin Lesion Segmentation via Iterative Stochastic Region Merging. IEEE Trans Inf Technol Biomed. 2011;15:929–36.
46. Mirikharaji Z, Abhishek K, Bissoto A, et al. A survey on deep learning for skin deficiency segmentation. Med Image Anal. 2023;88: 102863.
47. Lama N, Kasmi R, Hagerty JR, et al. ChimeraNet: U-Net for Hair Detection in Cosmoscopic Skin Lesion Images. J Digit Imaging. 2023;36(2):526–35.
48. Xu J, Wang X, Wang W, et al. PHCU Net: A parallel hierarchical cascade U-Net for skin loss segmentation. Biomedical Signal Processing and Control, 2023, 86 (Part B): 105262
49. Javed R, Rahim MSM, Saba T, et al. A comparative study of features selection for skin loss detection from Demoscopic images. Network Modeling Analysis in Health Informatics and Bioinformatics. 2020;9:1–13.
50. Rizzo M, Conati C, Jang D, et al. Cascading convolutional temporary color consistency. J Electron Imaging. 2023;32(1):1–13.
51. Land EH, McCann JJ. Lightness and retention theory. Josa. 1971;61(1):1–11.

52. Land EH. Recent advantages in retained theory and some implications for cortical calculations: color vision and the natural image. Proc Natl Acad Sci. 1983;80(16):5163–9.
53. Land EH. An alternative technique for the calculation of the designer in the retained theory of color vision. Proc Natl Acad Sci. 1986;83(10):3078–80.
54. Basri R, Jacobs DW. Lambertian reflection and linear subspaces IEEE transactions on pattern analysis machine intelligence. 2003;25(2):218–33.
55. Banić N. Lončarić S. Improving the white patch method by sampling. Paris:2014IEEE International Conference on Image Processing (ICIP), 2014: 605–609
56. Hordley S D, Finlayson G D. Re evaluating color consistency algorithms. Cambridge: Proceedings of the 17th International Conference on Pattern Recognition, 2004:76–79
57. Gijsenij A, Gevers T, Weijer JVD. Computational Color Consistency: Survey and Experiments. IEEE Trans Image Process. 2011;20(9):2475–89.
58. Van, De, Weijer, et al. Edge Based Color Consistency. IEEE Transactions on Image Processing, 2007, 16 (9): 2207–2214
59. Bianco S, Ciocca G, Cusano C, et al. Improving color consistency using indoor - outdoor image classification. IEEE Trans Image Process. 2008;17(12):2381–92.
60. Finlayson GD, Trezzi E. Shades of gray and color consistency. Scottsdale: Society for Imaging Science and Technology; 2004. p. 37–41.
61. Gijsenij A, Gevers T, Van De Weijer J. Improving color consistency by photographic edge weighting. IEEE Transactions on Pattern Analysis Machine Intelligence. 2011;34(5):918–29.
62. Forsyth DA. A novel algorithm for color consistency. Int J Comput Vision. 1990;5(1):5–35.
63. Finlayson G, Hordley S. Improving gamut mapping color consistency. IEEE Trans Image Process. 2000;9(10):1774–83.
64. Brainard DH, Freeman WT. Bayesian color consistency. JOSA A. 1997;14(7):1393–411.
65. Rizzi A, Gatta C, Marini D. A new algorithm for unsupervised global and local color correction. Pattern Recogn Lett. 2003;24(11):1663–77.
66. Babbar G, Bajaj R, Mittal N, et al. Hybrid model of alternating least squares and root polynomial technology for color correction. Soft Comput. 2023;27(8):4321–35.
67. Zhang W, Dong L, Xu W. Retinex inspired color correction and detailed preserved fusion for underwater image enhancement. Computers Electronics in Agriculture. 2022;192: 106585.
68. Barros F, Sousa PJ, Tavares PJ, et al. Digital image correlation through image registration in the frequency domain. The Journal of Strong Analysis for Engineering Design. 2018;53(8):575–83.
69. Ghani ASA. Image contrast enhancement using an integration of recursive overlapping contrast limited adaptive histogram specification and dual image wavelet fusion for the high visibility of deep underwater image. Ocean Eng. 2018;162:224–38.
70. Cheng D, Price B, Cohen S, et al. Effective learning based iluminant estimation using simple features. Boston: Proceedings of the IEEE conference on computer vision and pattern recognition, 2015: 1000–1008
71. Ma J, Fan X, Yang SX, et al. Contrast limited adaptive histogram equalization based fusion in YIQ and HSI color spaces for underwater image enhancement. International Journal of Pattern Recognition and Artistic Intelligence. 2018;32(07):1854018.
72. Wu S, Luo T, Jiang G, et al. A two-stage underwater enhancement network based on structure decomposition and characteristics of underwater imaging. IEEE Journal of Ocean Engineering. 2021;46(4):1213–27.
73. Jiang Y, Gong X, Liu D, et al. Enlightengan: Deep light enhancement without paid supervision. IEEE Trans Image Process. 2021;30:2340–9.
74. Liu X, Gao Z, Chen BM. MLFcGAN: Multiple feature fusion based conditional GAN for underwater image color correction. IEEE Geoscience Remote Sensing Letters. 2019;17(9):1488–92.
75. Chang S, Gao F, Zhang Q. Underwater Image Enhancement Method Based on Improved GAN and Physical Model. Electronics. 2023;12(13):2882.
76. Xue Z, Jiang X, Liu Q, et al. Global Local Facial Fusion Based GAN Generated Fake Face Detection. Sensors. 2023;23(2):616.

77. Shirai K, Baba T, Ono S, et al. Guided facial skin color correction. Signals. 2021;2(3):540–58.
78. Berbar MA. Skin color correction and faces detection techniques based on HSL and R color components. International Journal of Signal Imaging Systems Engineering. 2014;7(2):104–15.
79. Li X, Zhou F, Tan H, et al. Multi focus image fusion based on non-subsampled contourlet transformation and residual removal. Signal Process. 2021;184: 108062.
80. Wang L, Dou J, Qin P, et al. Multimodal medical image fusion based on non-subsampled shellet transformation and convolutional sparse representation. Multimedia Tools Applications. 2021;80:36401–21.
81. Li H, Wu X-J, Kittler J. MDLatLRR: A novel decomposition method for infrared and visible image fusion. IEEE Trans Image Process. 2020;29:4733–46.
82. Duarte AF, Sousa Pinto B, Azevedo LF, et al. Clinical ABCDE rule for early melanoma detection. Eur J Dermatol. 2021;31(6):771–8.
83. H Khan A, Iskandar D, Al Asad J F, et al. Classification of skin deficiency with hair and artifacts removing black hat pathology and total variation. International Journal of Computing and Digital Systems, 2021, 10:597–604
84. Schmid P. Segmentation of digitized dermal images by two dimensional color clustering. Signal Processing Laboratory, Swiss Federal Institute of Technology, Lausanne. 1999;18(2):164–71.
85. Nasonova A, Nasonov A, Krylov A, et al. Image warping in dermal image hair removal. PORTUGAL: Image Analysis and Recognition: 11th International Conference, 2014: 159–166
86. Saugeon PS, Guillod J, Third JP. Towards a computer aided diagnosis system for segmented skin lessons. Signal Processing Institute. 2003;27(1):65–78.
87. Kiani K, Sharafat AR. E-shaver: An improved DullRazor® for digitally removing dark and light colored hair in dermoscopic images. Cancer Control Research. 2011;41(3):139–45.
88. Boris D, Kowalska P, Frackiewicz M, et al. A simple hair removal algorithm from dermoscopic images. Grenada: Bioinformatics and Biomedical Engineering: Third International Conference, 2015: 262–273
89. T L. V. N, R. G, et al. Dullrazor: a software approach to hair removal from images. Cancer Control Research, 1997, 27 (6): 533–543
90. Nguyen N H, Lee T K, Atkins M S. Segmentation of light and dark hair in dermoscopic images: a hybrid approach using a universal kernel. San Diego: Medical Imaging 2010: Image Processing 2010: 1436–1443
91. Abbas Q, Celebi ME, García IF. Hair removal methods: a comparative study for dermoscopic images. Biomedical Signal Processing Control. 2011;6(4):395–404.
92. Huang A, Kwan S-Y, Chang W-Y, et al. A robust hair segmentation and removal approach for clinical images of skin regions. Osaka: 2013 35th Annual International Conference of the IEEE Engineering in Medicine and Biology Society (EMBC), 2013: 3315–3318
93. Bibilloni P, Gonz á lez Hilalgo M, Massanet S. Skin hair removal in dermoscopic images using soft color morphology. Vienna: Artistic Intelligence in Medicine: 16th Conference on Artistic Intelligence in Medicine, 2017: 322–326
94. Satheesha TY, Satyanarayana D, Giriprasad MN. A Pixel Interpolation Technique for curved hair removal in skin images to support melanoma detection. Journal of Theoretical Applied Information Technology. 2014;70(3):559–65.
95. Koehoorn J, Sobiecki A C, Boda D, et al. Automated digital hair removal by threshold decomposition and morphological analysis. Reykjavik: Mathematical Philosophy and Its Applications to Signal and Image Processing: 12th International Symposium, 2015: 15–26
96. Mirzaalian H, Lee TK, Hamarneh G. Hair enhancement in dermoscopic images using dual channel quantization tuition filters and MRF based multilingual optimization. IEEE Trans Image Process. 2014;23(12):5486–96.
97. Mahmood D a F, Mahmood H A. Artifact Removal from Skin Dermoscopy Imagesto Support Automated Melanoma Diagnosis. Al Rafidain Engineering Journal (AREJ), 2015, 23 (5): 22–30

98. Das P, Gangopadyay M. Removal of hair particles from skin disease images using pixel based approach. International Journal of Computer Science and Information Technologies. 2015;6(5):15–6.
99. Medioni G, Lee M-S, Tang C-K. A computational framework for segmentation and grouping. Amsterdam: Elsevier; 2000.
100. Tong W-S. Tang C-K Robust estimation of adaptive tensors of curvature by tensor voting. IEEE Trans Pattern Anal Mach Intell. 2005;27(3):434–49.
101. Eggersmann R, Stainier L, Ortiz M, et al. Model free data driven computational mechanics enhanced by tensor voting. Comput Methods Appl Mech Eng. 2021;373: 113499.
102. Liu H. Xiao G-F Remote sensing image registration based on improved KAZE and BRIEF descriptor. International Journal of Automation Computing. 2020;17(4):588–98.
103. Loss LA, Bebis G, Parvin B. Interactive tensor voting for perceptual grouping of ill defined curved structures. Signal Processing Laboratory, Swiss Federal Institute of Technology, Lausanne. 2011;30(8):1503–13.
104. Yao F. Damaged region filling by improved crime image painting algorithm for thangka. Information Processing and Visualization Technology. 2019;22(6):13683–91.
105. Ouattara N, Loum GL, Pandry GK, et al. A new image painting approach based on Criminisi algorithm. Int J Adv Comput Sci Appl. 2019;10(6):423–33.
106. Xu Z, Sun J. Image painting by patch promotion using patch sparsity. IEEE Trans Image Process. 2010;19(5):1153–65.
107. Hesabi S, Mahdavi Amiri N. A modified patch promotion based image painting using patch sparsity. Shiraz: The 16th CSI International Symposium on Artistic Intelligence and Signal Processing (AISP 2012), 2012: 043–048
108. Criminisi A, Perez P, Toyama K. Object removal by exemplar based repainting. MADISON: 2003 IEEE Computer Society Conference on Computer Vision and Pattern Recognition, 2003 Proceedings, 2003: II-II
109. Jin D, Bai X. Patch party based image painting through a facet produced directional derivative. IEEE Transactions on Circuits Systems for Video Technology. 2018;29(5):1310–24.
110. Zeng C, Wang M. Fast converting image painting method based on BSCB model. Journal of Algorithms Computational Technology. 2009;3(3):331–41.
111. Chen Y, Liu L, Tao J, et al. The improved image painting algorithm via encoder and similarity constraint. Vis Comput. 2021;37:1691–705.
112. Li K, Wei Y, Yang Z, et al. Image painting algorithm based on TV model and evolutionary algorithm. Soft Comput. 2016;20:885–93.
113. Chan TF, Shen J. Nontext painting by curvature driven diffusion. Journal of Visual Communication Image Representation. 2001;12(4):436–49.
114. Liang Z, Ding X, Jin J, et al. A Color Cast Image Enhancement Method Based on Affine Transform in Poor Visible Conditions. IEEE Geosci Remote Sens Lett. 2022;19:1–5.
115. Shangguan Jintai Research on Several Issues in Image Registration. Chengdu: Sichuan University Press, 2020
116. Chen K, Ren Z, Yan F, et al. Quantum implementation of image registration. Quantum Information Processing, 2023, 22 (2)
117. Zhao M, Ma L, Jia X, et al. Graphreg: Dynamic point cloud registration with geometry aware graph signal processing. IEEE Trans Image Process. 2022;31:7449–64.
118. Duan J, Jia X, Bartlett J, et al. Arbitrary Order Total Variation for Deformable Image Registration. Pattern Recogn. 2023;137: 109318.
119. Ghaffari A, Fatemizadeh E. Image registration based on low rank matrix: Rank regulated SSD. Signal Processing Laboratory, Swiss Federal Institute of Technology, Lausanne. 2017;37(1):138–50.
120. Zheng Q, Wang Q, Ba X, et al. A medical image registration method based on progressive images. Computational Mathematical Methods in Medicine. 2021;2021:1–9.
121. Darkner S, Vidarte JD, Lauze F. First Order Locally Orderless Registration. Lect Notes Comput Sci. 2021;12679:177–88.

122. Jia W. A novel image registration control system based on improved composite metric entropy function in color printing. Multimedia Tools Applications. 2020;79:9225–36.
123. Gong M, Zhao S, Jiao L, et al. A novel coat to fine scheme for automatic image registration based on SIFT and multiple information. IEEE transactions on geoscience remote sensing. 2013;52(7):4328–38.
124. Gharbia R, Ahmed S A, Hassanien A E. Remote sensing image registration based on particle swarm optimization and multiple information. Kaliani: Information Systems Design and Intelligent Applications: Proceedings of Second International Conference INDIA 2015, 2015: 399–408
125. Chen, Li, Zhao, et al. Medium low resolution multisource remote sensing image registration based on SIFT and robust regional multiple information. International Journal of Remote Sensing, 2018, 39 (10): 3215–3242
126. Oliveira FP, Pataky TC, Tavares JMR. Registration of pedestrian image data in the frequency domain. Computer methods in biomedical engineering. 2010;13(6):731–40.
127. Huang J, An D, Luo Y, et al. A Registration Method for Dual Frequency, High Spatial Resolution SAR I images. Remote Sensing. 2022;14(10):2509.
128. Qu X, Huo H, Lian S, et al. A novel frequency domain iterative image registration algorithm based on local region extraction. Mathematical Problems in Engineering, 2015, 2015
129. Yu X, Lyu Z, Hu D, et al. Scale invariant feature transformation based on the frequency spectrum and the grid for remote sensing image registration. GIScience&Remote Sensing. 2013;50(5):543–61.
130. Dellinger F, Delon J, Gousseau Y, et al. SAR SIFT: A SIFT-LIKE Algorithm for SAR images. IEEE Transactions on Geoscience Remote Sensing. 2013;53(1):453–66.
131. Sun J, Lu H, Liu X. Saliency region detection based on Markov absorption probabilities. IEEE Trans Image Process. 2015;24(5):1639–49.
132. Chanchlani MP, Khambete M. A Novel Speed-up Feature Matching Algorithm for Image Registration using SUSAN and RANSAC. IJEAT. 2013;33(360):2026–35.
133. Fang Y, Liu W, Gao M, et al. Improved accurate image registration algorithm based on FREAK descriptor. Journal of Computer Applications. 2016;36(12):3402.
134. Schwind P, D’Angelo P. Evaluating the application of BRISK for the geometric registration of remote sensing images. Remote Sending Letters. 2015;6(9):677–86.
135. Zhang Z, Wang L, Zheng W, et al. Endoscope image mosaic based on pyramid ORB. Biomedical Signal Processing Control. 2022;71: 103261.
136. Zhang W, Zhao Y. An improved SIFT algorithm for registration between SAR and optical images. Sci Rep. 2023;13(1):6346.
137. Ordóñez Á, Acción Á, Argüello F, et al. HSI MSER: Hyperspectral Image Registration Algorithm Based on MSER and SIFT. IEEE Journal of Selected Topics in Applied Earth Observations Remote Sensing. 2021;14:12061–72.
138. Divya S, Paul S, Pati UC. Structure tensor based SIFT algorithm for SAR image registration. IET Image Process. 2020;14(5):929–38.
139. Lowe DG. Distinctive image features from scale invariant keypoints. Int J Comput Vision. 2004;60:91–110.
140. Bin J, Zhang H, Bahrami Z, et al. The registration of visible and thermal images through multi-objective optimization. MOVEJ Analytic, 2023, 95 (C): 186–198
141. Chum O, Matas J. Matching with PROSAC progressive sample consensus. San Diego: 2005 IEEE Computer Society Conference on Computer Vision and Pattern Recognition (CVPR’05) 2005: 220–226

# Chapter 2
# Color Correction Models

## 2.1 Introduction

Dermatoscopy is a non-invasive diagnostic tool, whose application scope has gradually expanded from the earliest diagnosis and classification of the melanoma to the diagnosis and classification of the pigmentary diseases such as nevi, seborrheic keratosis, basal cell carcinoma, vascular tumors, and hemorrhagic lesions. Dermatoscopy can reduce the reflection interference of light, magnify the local lesion region up to 25–150 times or even larger, and observe the skin structure and morphology at the junction of the epidermis, epidermis, and dermis, and even the surface layer of the epidermis. Various structures, such as pigment network structure, dot-like structure, pebble-like structure, "blue white" veil, degenerative structure, comma shaped blood vessels, and other typical skin disease symptoms of ZA can be observed [1, 2]. Due to deviations in daytime temperatures, light angles, photography parameters, and the refraction and reflection interferences of artificial light sources under different polarized light conditions, there are many color deviations in dermoscopic images on different environments.

Typical dermoscopic image color deviations include image blueness caused by the lack of compensation for the color brought by artificial light sources (see Fig. 2.1a1). Due to the dark color of the lesion location, there is a high light overexposure in the dermatoscope, that is, the high light region is too bright, and easily leads to severe loss of image details (see Fig. 2.1a2); While insufficient exposure leads to insufficient brightness of the image, and further an overall darkening of the image (see Fig. 2.1a3). In addition, due to the patient's frequent scratching the skin or rupture of capillaries, the local skin color turns red, which is not a color characteristic of the skin disease itself [3] (the skin with pathological changes such as red, purple, localized hardening, diffuse hardening, and so on are respectively shown in Fig. 2.1b). Compared to other medical images, the color features of lesion regions in dermatoscopic images are influenced by the patient's skin color [4, 5]. There are significant deviations in skin color among different races, and even within the same race, patients of different



S. Guo et al., *Computer-Aided Intelligent Diagnosis of Skin Melanoma*,
https://doi.org/10.1007/978-981-96-6135-0_2

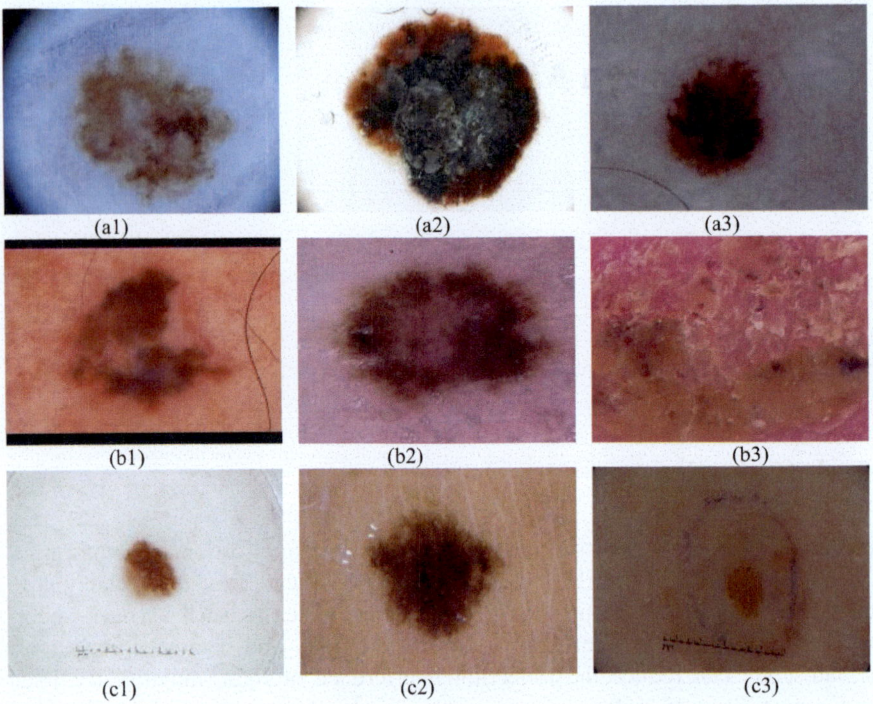


**Fig. 2.1** Color deviations of dermoscopic images (**a** color deviation caused by light source and equipment, **b** abnormal skin color of patients, **c** different skin color deviation of patients)

genders and ages (the manifestation of lesion regions in the white human being, the yellow human being, and the brown human being is shown in Fig. 2.1c, respectively). Therefore, it is necessary to correct the color of the dermoscopic image in order to eliminate any abnormal color interference in the dermoscopic image as much as possible.

The color correction of dermoscopic images requires certain assumptions on the color constancy [6, 7], and then the gamma correction and so on [8] is used to adjust the color or the brightness of the image. How to construct a suitable objective function and solve it is a key issue in the color correction of dermoscopic image [9]. The optimal solution of the objective function requires the objective function to be convex [10], and the presence of multiple constraints during the correction process also brings the solution of the objective function more complex [11]. Different constraint conditions during the image correction process are separately solved, and then the fused solutions can effectively meet the quality requirements for correction results in different scenarios [12, 13]. In response to the above issues, a method based on gamma correction and multi-scale image fusion is proposed, i.e. constraint conditions are constructed based on the average pixel value and the average brightness of the image, and the unconstrained color difference criterion is transformed into solving the objective function with constraints. By smoothing the objective function and using the Lagrangian dual method, the constrained optimization problem is transformed into a convex optimization problem of the objective function; Then, the objective function is solved using the Newton iteration method, and the initial value dependency in the Newton iteration method is solved using the binary method to obtain the preliminary image correction results; Finally, the result of dermoscopic image color correction is obtained through the image fusion.

## 2.2 Color Correction Model with Gamma Correction and Multi-scale Image Fusion

The color correction model based on gamma correction and multi-scale image fusion includes a gamma correction model based on Newton iteration method and a multi-scale image fusion model, which respectively solve the objective function with the color constraints, and average unchanged brightness; The key scientific issue is to ensure the quality and clarity of fused images by integrating detailed texture features and basic color brightness information from multi-scale images. The framework of the overall model is shown in Fig. 2.2.

### *2.2.1 The Gamma Color Correction Model*

The gamma correction is a common nonlinear method, which adjusts the image brightness, and achieves the goal of correcting image color by performing exponential operations on each pixel [14]. The transformation function for the gamma correction is:

$$\tilde{f}_i(x, y) = f_i^{\gamma_i}(x, y) \tag{2.1}$$

where $\tilde{f}_i(x, y)$ represents the image value of the $i$th channel pixel $(x, y)$ after correction. The abnormal color images often have mismatched pixel distributions between different color channels, which results in the abnormal visual effects. The color correction can be achieved by reducing the distribution color deviations among different color channels. Let the maximum difference between the average value of each color channel and the total average value of the three channels as the color difference criterion, the objective function is defined as follows:

$$\Delta(\gamma_r, \gamma_g, \gamma_b) = \max\left\{\left|\overline{\tilde{f}}_r(x, y) - \overline{\tilde{M}}\right|, \left|\overline{\tilde{f}}_g(x, y) - \overline{\tilde{M}}\right|, \left|\overline{\tilde{f}}_b(x, y) - \overline{\tilde{M}}\right|\right\} \tag{2.2}$$

where, $\gamma_r, \gamma_g, \gamma_b$ are the correction coefficients for each channel, $M = (f_r(x, y) + f_g(x, y) + f_b(x, y))/3$, $\overline{\tilde{f}}_r(x, y)$, $\overline{\tilde{f}}_g(x, y)$ and $\overline{\tilde{f}}_b(x, y)$ respectively represent the pixel means of the corrected color channel.

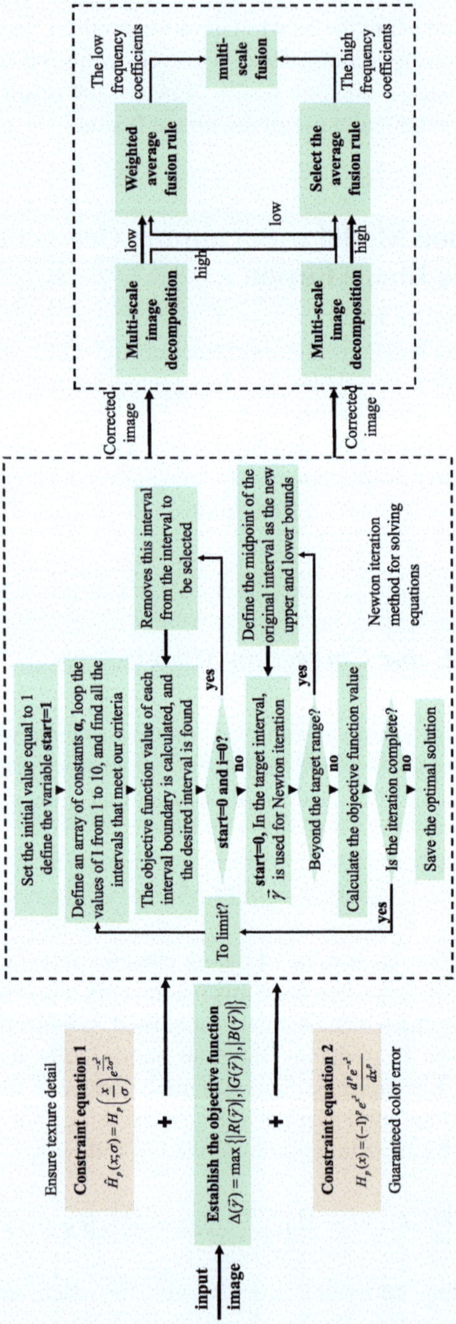


**Fig. 2.2** The framework for color correction of skin disease images

The objective function for adjusting color differences is defined as:

$$\Delta(\gamma_r, \gamma_g, \gamma_b) = \max\left\{\begin{array}{l} \left|2\bar{\bar{f}}_r^{\gamma_r}(x, y) - \bar{\bar{f}}_g^{\gamma_g}(x, y) - \bar{\bar{f}}_b^{\gamma_b}(x, y)\right|, \\ \left|-\bar{\bar{f}}_r^{\gamma_r}(x, y) + 2\bar{\bar{f}}_g^{\gamma_g}(x, y) - \bar{\bar{f}}_b^{\gamma_b}(x, y)\right|, \\ \left|-\bar{\bar{f}}_r^{\gamma_r}(x, y) - \bar{\bar{f}}_g^{\gamma_g}(x, y) + 2\bar{\bar{f}}_b^{\gamma_b}(x, y)\right| \end{array}\right\} \tag{2.3}$$

And let $g_g(\vec{\gamma}) = -\bar{\bar{f}}_r^{\gamma_r}(x, y) + 2\bar{\bar{f}}_g^{\gamma_g}(x, y) - \bar{\bar{f}}_b^{\gamma_b}(x, y)$, $g_r(\vec{\gamma}) = 2\bar{\bar{f}}_r^{\gamma_r}(x, y) - \bar{\bar{f}}_g^{\gamma_g}(x, y) - \bar{\bar{f}}_b^{\gamma_b}(x, y)$, $g_b(\vec{\gamma}) = -\bar{\bar{f}}_r^{\gamma_r}(x, y) - \bar{\bar{f}}_g^{\gamma_g}(x, y) + 2\bar{\bar{f}}_b^{\gamma_b}(x, y)$, , then the objective function (2.3) can be rewritten as:

$$\Delta(\vec{\gamma}) = \max\left\{|g_r(\vec{\gamma})|, \left|g_g(\vec{\gamma})\right|, |g_b(\vec{\gamma})|\right\} \tag{2.4}$$

When each gamma coefficient is set to zero or infinity, the color difference can be reduced to zero, and the image is either completely white or completely black. However, this gamma value is not the objective solution, so the objective function cannot be directly solved. In order to preserve a unique solution and ensure that the image is not distorted during the correction process, it is necessary to add constraints to the optimization, and the solved problem becomes:

$$\min \quad \Delta(\vec{\gamma}) \quad \text{s.t.} \quad \tilde{Y}(\gamma) = Y_0 \tag{2.5}$$

where $Y_0 = Y(1)$, $\tilde{Y}(\gamma)$ is the constructed constraint condition.

It is well-known that the objective function is a nonlinear equation and not a smooth function. In order to make the objective function differentiable, some improvements have been done, for example, the square function and the normalized Log-Sum-Exp function are correspondingly used instead of the absolute value function and the maximum value function,

$$\Delta(\vec{\gamma}) = \ln\Big(\exp(g_r^2(\vec{\gamma})) + \exp\Big(g_g^2(\vec{\gamma})\Big) + \exp(g_b^2(\vec{\gamma})) - 2\Big) \tag{2.6}$$

where the constant term is guaranteed through $LSE(0, 0, 0) = \ln(1) = 0$.

When one of $\gamma_r, \gamma_g, \gamma_b$ is fixed, a nonlinear equation/system can be constructed by assuming that the color difference of the corrected image is 0, and further calculates the two remaining gamma corrected parameters. So, whether there is a unique solution for (2.5) is transformed into whether there is a unique solution for $\tilde{Y}_r(\gamma_r) = Y_0$.

If the optimal solution $\gamma_r^*$ is taken as the root of the above equation, the optimal solutions $\gamma_b$ and $\gamma_g$ can be transformed into their own solving problems. If the constraint equation is a strictly monotonically decreasing continuous function on $\gamma_r$, when $\gamma_r = 0$, it reaches to the maximum value of 1, and when $\gamma_r \to \infty$, it approaches to the minimum value of 0. Due to the initial constraint equation taking values between 0 and 1, according to the mean value theorem, when the monotonically decreasing function $\gamma_r$ satisfies $\tilde{Y}_r(\gamma_r) = Y_0$, there must be a unique solution $\gamma_r^*$, and further $\gamma_g^*$ and $\gamma_b^*$ are obtained.

During the optimization process of the objective function, the Lagrangian duality method is used to transform the constrained optimization into a convex optimization without constraints or with simpler constraints. The Lagrangian dual equation is given by (2.7):

$$L(\vec{\gamma}, v) = \Delta(\vec{\gamma}) + v\big(\tilde{Y}(\vec{\gamma}) - Y_0\big) \tag{2.7}$$

And its associated dual function is given by Eq. (2.8)

$$h(v) = \inf_{\vec{\gamma}}\big(\Delta(\vec{\gamma}) + v\tilde{Y}(\vec{\gamma})\big) - vY_0 \tag{2.8}$$

Due to $\Delta(\vec{\gamma}) > 0$ and the uniqueness of the solution, the equation $h(v)$ approaches zero when $\vec{\gamma}$ approaches infinity and $\Delta(0) = 0$. In general, it is necessary to construct constraints $h(v)$ equal to 1 when $h(v) = 0$, and $h(v)$ close to 0 when $\vec{\gamma} \to \infty$. It means that the infimum of the dual function $h(v)$ is determined by the corresponding constraint equations, for example, if the sign of the dual function is determined by $v \geq 0$, then the infimum is obtained in any direction $\vec{\gamma}$ when $\vec{\gamma} \to \infty$. If $v < 0$, then the infimum is realized at $\vec{\gamma} = 0$, and then the first term of Eq. (2.8) is zero, and its second term reaches to the maximum value 1. If $v$ is negative, then its infimum is $v$ itself.

In short, the above dual problem is given by (2.9):

$$g(v) = \begin{cases} -vY_0 & \mathit{if}\ v \geq 0 \\ v(1 - Y_0) & \mathit{if}\ v < 0 \end{cases} \tag{2.9}$$

By analyzing formula (2.9), it can be shown that the objective function is a strong duality, and both the maximum value of the dual problem and the minimum value of its original problem are zero. Therefore, to ensure the existence of the solution of the objective function, it is necessary to ensure that the initial values of the constraint equations are finite in any image.

Note: (1) It is proposed to construct two different constraint conditions based on the average pixel values of the image and the average brightness, respectively, and to transform the unconstrained color difference criterion into optimizing the constrained objective function. After obtaining different correction results based on the above two types of constraints, the processed images will further be fused to enhance the quality of image correction.

(2) It is well-known that solving the objective function with initial states is a non-convex problem, which is transformed into a convex optimization by smoothing the above objective function and further using the Lagrangian duality method.

In fact, many standard optimization methods can be applied to solve smooth objective functions $\Delta(\vec{\gamma})$. However, due to the fact that the objective function $\vec{\gamma}$

will inevitably approach a minimum or a stationary point when its coefficients all approach infinity, it is highly likely that many descent methods often tend towards these infinite minimum values. Therefore, the constraint term is added as a quadratic penalty term to the above objective function.

The relevant minimization process is calculated during each step by Eq. (2.10):

$$\vec{\gamma}_{k+1} = \arg\min \Delta(\vec{\gamma}) + \frac{\mu_k}{2}\left(\tilde{Y}(\vec{\gamma}) - Y_0\right)^2 \tag{2.10}$$

After a series of improvements, the objective function can be effectively solved using the Newton's method. It is well known that the Newton's method clearly depends on the initial value $\vec{\gamma}_0$ and $\mu$. For the smaller values $\mu$, the penalty term is often insufficient to force the constraint term to reach to the true minimum, and the solution will drift towards infinity. Considering that the binary method is easy to determine the existence of solutions, which is used to optimize selecting the initial value of the Newton's method, i.e. the domain of the objective function is divided into several regions and the binary method is used to find a possible interval where the solution may exist. The boundary value of the obtained interval is defined as the initial value, and the Newton iterative formula is applied to find the optimal solution of the objective function.

The important calculation steps are listed as follows.

Step 1: A $n$-dimensional constant array $[\alpha_1, \alpha_2 \cdots \alpha_n]$ is defined to calculate the corresponding objective function value, where $[\alpha_1, \alpha_n]$ is the defined domain of the objective function. Based on the binary approach, if

$$\Delta(\vec{\gamma}_{k+1}) \cdot \Delta(\vec{\gamma}_k) < 0 \tag{2.11}$$

Then, there exists a solution within the interval $\left[\gamma_0\alpha_i, \gamma_0\alpha_{i+1}\right]$. The value of $i$ is traversed from 1 to $n$, and all intervals that satisfy the conditions are obtained.

Step 2: The corresponding target color difference function for each interval boundary $\left[\alpha_i, \alpha_{i+1}\right]$ is calculated, and the lowest image color difference interval corresponding to their boundary values is found.

Step 3: Within the target interval, it starts from the midpoint of the interval, and iterates according to the Newton's iterative formula until a target value $\vec{\gamma}$ that meets all conditions is obtained. When the midpoint of the target interval is not the target value, it needs to define the midpoint of the original interval as a new boundary and keeps the other boundary unchanged. Thereafter, Step 3 is repeated within the newly defined target interval.

Note: It is proposed that the domain of the objective function is divided into several regions and the binary method is used to find the possible interval for the objective solution, thereby the initial value dependence of Newton's iteration method is solved.

### 2.2.2 Multi-scale Image Fusion Model

In order to fuse the correction results under different constraints to obtain a more ideal processed image, it is necessary to perform two-dimensional orthogonal wavelet decomposition on the original image, adopt different fusion strategies to complete the fusion of different frequency components, and make the fused image retain the significant features of the initial correction image in different frequency domains as much as possible.

**Image decomposition and reconstruction**

The wavelet transform can decompose an original image into the different frequency-domain components. Through image decomposition and reconstruction, the desired feature distribution can simultaneously be obtained in the time–frequency domain [15]. There exists a multi-resolution series $V_j^2(j \in Z)$ in space $L^2(R^2)$, whose orthonormal basis functions are composed of a scale function system $\{\varphi_{j,m_1,m_2}|(m_1, m_2) \in Z^2\}$ and a wavelet function system $\left\{\psi^{\varepsilon}_{j,m_1,m_2}|(m_1, m_2) \in Z^2; \varepsilon = 1, 2, 3\right\}$, respectively, while the low-pass filter $\{h(k)\}$ and the high pass filter $\{g(k)\}$ are the coefficients of the dual scale equations of the above two types of orthonormal basis functions.

For pending the original image $f(x, y) \in L^2(R \times R)$, two-dimensional orthogonal wavelet decomposition equations are as follows:

$$
\begin{aligned}
C_{1,j}(x, y) &= \sum_{k,l} h(k - 2x)h(l - 2y)C_j(k, l) \\
D_{1,j}(x, y) &= \sum_{k,l} g(k - 2x)h(l - 2y)C_j(k, l) \\
D_{2,j}(x, y) &= \sum_{k,l} h(k - 2x)g(l - 2y)C_j(k, l) \\
D_{3,j}(x, y) &= \sum_{k,l} g(k - 2x)g(l - 2y)C_j(k, l)
\end{aligned}
\tag{2.12}
$$

where, $C_1(x, y)$ represents the low-frequency component of the image, $D_{i,j}(x, y)(i = 1, 2, 3)$ does the high-frequency components of the image in the vertical, the horizontal, and the diagonal, respectively.

After processing the components in various directions of the decomposed image, Eq. (2.13) can be used to reconstruct the complete image.

$$
\begin{aligned}
C_j(x, y) = &\sum_{k,l} C_1(k, l)h(x - 2k)h(y - 2l) \\
&+ \sum_{k,l} D_1(k, l)g(x - 2k)h(y - 2l)
\end{aligned}
$$

$$+\sum_{k,l} D_2(k,l)h(x-2k)g(y-2l)$$
$$+\sum_{k,l} D_3(k,l)g(x-2k)g(y-2l) \tag{2.13}$$

After using Eq. (2.12) to perform wavelet decomposition on a certain dermatoscope image, the results are shown in Fig. 2.3, from which it is clear for the high-frequency and low-frequency component information of the image. The high-frequency component of an image, which contains many information such as the edges (contours), the details, and the textures of the image, mainly refers to the contour and the texture information of the lesion region in the image, and is the main basis for disease recognition. Therefore, for the fusion of high-frequency components, the local energy is adopted to reflect some information contained in the images, and simultaneously, the different fusion criteria are selected. Through smooth intensity (brightness/grayscale) transformations, the low-frequency components of an image include the pixel points, which are mainly comprehensive measures of the entire dermatoscope image intensity. As is the main content of color correction, the weighted optimized artificial fish swarm fusion algorithm is adopted to ensure the fusion quality of the image.

**High Frequency Component Fusion**

Assuming that the two processed images obtained from the original image $f(x, y)$ after correction are decomposed into the high-frequency components $D_{i,A}(x, y)$ and $D_{i,B}(x, y)$, $i = 1, 2, 3$ respectively through the wavelet transform, which respectively represent the high-frequency components of the processed image on the horizontal, the vertical, and the diagonal.

The local area energy $E_{i,A}$, $E_{i,B}$ of the high-frequency components of the processed image can be obtained using the wavelet coefficient matrix, whose calculation equations are

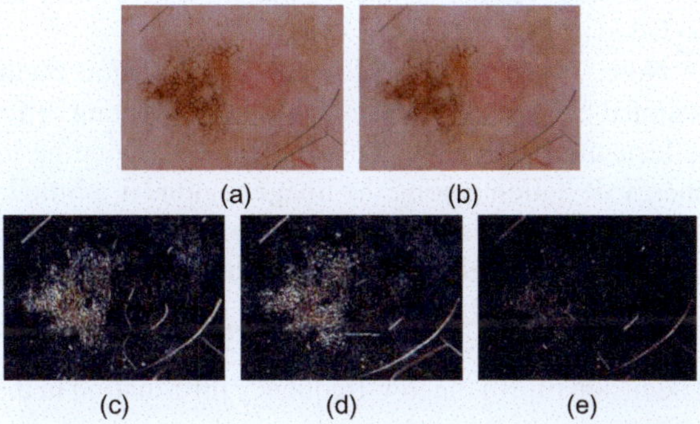


**Fig. 2.3** Wavelet decomposition of dermoscopic image (**a** original image, **b** low-frequency component, **c** vertical high-frequency component, **d** horizontal high-frequency component, **e** diagonal high-frequency component)

$$E_{i,w}(x,y)=\sum_{x\in L}\sum_{y\in K}W(x',y')\left[D_{j,\omega}(x+x',y+y')\right]^2 \quad w=A \text{ or } B \tag{2.14}$$

where, $E_{i,w}(x, y)$ represents the energy of the image $w$, $(x, y)$ does as the center and $L$, $K$ does the length and width of the local region. $W(x', y')$ does the corresponding wavelet coefficient.

And further the corresponding matching degree of the region $A$, $B$ can be designed as

$$M_{i,w}(x,y)=\frac{2\sum_{x\in L}\sum_{y\in K}W(x',y')D_{i,A}(x+x',y+y')D_{i,B}(x+x',y+y')}{E_{i,A}(x,y)+E_{i,B}(x,y)} \tag{2.15}$$

and the matching degree of regions is used to classify through a threshold $\tau\in[0.5,1]$ as follows.

If $M_{i,w}(x, y)\geq\tau$, then

$$D_{i,F}(x,y)=W_{i,L}(x,y)D_{i,A}(x,y)+W_{i,S}(x,y)D_{i,B}(x,y) \tag{2.16}$$

$$W_{i,S}(x,y)=\frac{1}{2}\left(1-\frac{1-M_{i,AB}(x,y)}{1-\delta}\right) \tag{2.17}$$

$$W_{i,L}(x,y)=1-W_{i,S}(x,y) \tag{2.18}$$

otherwise

$$D_{i,F}(x,y)=\begin{cases}D_{i,A}(x,y) & E_{i,A}(x,y)\geq E_{i,B}(x,y)\\ D_{i,B}(x,y) & E_{i,A}(x,y)<E_{i,B}(x,y)\end{cases} \tag{2.19}$$

where, $D_{i,F}(x, y)$ denotes the high-frequency component of the fused image.

For the fused image, the coefficient arrays of the high-frequency components can be listed as Eqs. (2.14)–(2.18).

Note: An adaptive matching degree fusion method is proposed based on the regional energy, i.e. the matching degree among different images to a certain extent reflects their energy deviation in the corresponding regions. For example, when the energy deviation among the image regions is a little large, the image pixels with the higher energy are selected as the interested points. Otherwise, the final fusion result is achieved through the above weighted methods.

**Low-frequency Components Optimization Fusion**

The fusion rule of the low-frequency information in the images is designed as follows

$$C_{i,F}(i,j)=a\cdot C_{i,A}(i,j)+b\cdot C_{i,B}(i,j) \tag{2.20}$$

where $C_{i,F}(x, y)$ is the low-frequency component of the fused image, $C_{i,A}(x, y)$ and $C_{i,B}(x, y)$ are the low-frequency components of the images $A$, $B$ to be fused, $a$ and $b$ are the weight parameters. The resolution is held as much as possible, and simultaneously more sub-image information is kept for the low-frequency component of the fused image. Combining the cross entropy and the average gradient as the fused image objective function, the artificial fish swarm algorithm is used to optimize the weight parameters to obtain the ideal fusion parameters.

The proposed image fusion objective function is defined as follows

$$H = AG - \overline{CH} \tag{2.21}$$

where $AG$ is the average gradient of the image, and the $\overline{CH}$ does the overall cross entropy of the fused image and the original image.

$AG$ and $\overline{CH}$ are calculated using Eqs. (2.22) and (2.23), respectively.

$$AG = \frac{\sum_{i=1}^{m-1}\sum_{j=1}^{n-1}\sqrt{\frac{(C_{i,F}(i+1,j)-C_{i,F}(i,j))^2+(C_{i,F}(i,j+1)-C_{i,F}(i,j))^2}{2}}}{(m-1)(n-1)} \tag{2.22}$$

$$\overline{CH} = \sqrt{\left(CH_P^2 + CH_Q^2\right)/2} \tag{2.23}$$

where $m$, $n$ represents the length and width of the image, respectively, $CH_P$, $CH_Q$ represent the cross entropies of the original image $P$ and the fused image $Q$, respectively.

And $CH_j$, $(j = P, Q)$ is calculated as follows:

$$CH_j = \sum_{i=1}^{L} p_i \ln(p_i / q_i) \tag{2.24}$$

where $p_i$ and $q_i$ represent the ratio of the pixel number of $i$th region and the total pixel number of the image, respectively, and $L$ does the grayscale level of the image.

Note: For the image fusing, the larger the average gradient, the higher the image clarity and the fused quality, while the smaller the cross entropy of the fused image, the better the fused quality.

In the process of optimizing the weight parameters of the artificial fish swarm algorithm [16], each artificial fish updates its own state by executing different functions such as foraging, crowding, swallowing, etc. And those parameters that can be adjusted in the above algorithm include the maximum number of iterations $g_{\max}$, the number of artificial fish $N$, the artificial fish state parameters $X$, the step size $S$, the field of view $V$, the maximum number of artificial fish attempts $t$, the crowding factor parameters $\delta$, and the perceptual distance *visual*. However, the above-mentioned artificial fish swarm algorithm has some shortcomings such as the complex solving process and the long calculation time in practice.

Therefore, the following necessary adjustments and improvements are proposed:

(1) Some adjustments on the artificial fish visual field and the step size

For the traditional corresponding algorithms, the search field of view and the step size of the artificial fish swarm are fixed. In order to ensure that relevant algorithms have strong global search ability and will not directly fall into local optima, it is necessary to set the field of view and the step size to larger scopes. However, those will increase the complexity of the algorithm and simultaneously increase its running time to a certain extent. Therefore, the search field of view $V$ and the step size $S$ of the artificial fish are set as follows

$$V = \left[ (V_{\max} - V_{\min}) \frac{1}{\sqrt{2\pi}\sigma} e^{-\frac{(g/g_{\max})^2}{2\sigma^2}} + V_{\min} \right] Rand(0, 1) \tag{2.25}$$

$$S = \left[ (S_{\max} - S_{\min}) \frac{1}{\sqrt{2\pi}\sigma} e^{-\frac{(g/g_{\max})^2}{2\sigma^2}} + S_{\min} \right] Rand(0, 1) \tag{2.26}$$

where, $V_{\max}$ and $V_{\min}$ respectively represent the superior and inferior limits of the artificial fish's field of view; $S_{\max}$ and $S_{\min}$ respectively represent the superior and inferior limits of the step size for artificial fish; $g$ does the current number of iterations; $\sigma$ does the standard deviation of a normal distribution.

Note: The improved artificial fish search field of view and the step size can enable the improved artificial fish swarm algorithm to have a larger field of view and a larger step size in the early stages of iteration, and easily search for all possible regions as quickly as possible. In the later stage of iteration, more accurate solutions are obtained by reducing the step size and the field of view, while the accuracy of the proposed algorithm is increased.

(2) Mutation strategies

During algorithm iteration and optimization, the artificial fish swarm may be trapped in local optimal solutions, and mutation strategies are introduced to avoid the above phenomenon as much as possible. In the practical operation, if the position of the artificial fish swarm does not change continuously for at least five times, a mutation operation is performed on the artificial fish swarm. Assuming that the probability of the artificial fish variation is $P_m$ and its total number is $mP_m$, and when an artificial fish swarm undergoes a certain mutations, its states update as Eq. (2.27).

$$x_i^{t+1} = \begin{cases} a + (b - x_i^t) & x_i^t \geq (a+b)/2 \\ b - (x_i^t - a) & x_i^t < (a+b)/2 \end{cases} \tag{2.27}$$

where, $x_i^t$ is the $i$th state of the artificial fish school at time $t$, and the range of independent variables $x$ is $[a, b]$.

(3) Swallowing behaviors

In order to accelerate the running speed of the artificial fish swarm algorithm, when the number of iterations reaches to half of the maximum, the artificial fishes whose states have always exceeded the set values are discarded. At this time, the sum of artificial fishes is defined as $n - 1$.

The flowchart of the improved artificial fish swarm algorithm is shown in Fig. 2.4.

## 2.3 Experimental Simulation

In the experimental section, two groups of experiments are set up to evaluate the effectiveness of the improved algorithm. The first group demonstrates the effectiveness of color correction and the improved image fusion algorithm through five sets of dermoscopic images. The second group utilizes more diverse types of dermoscopic images to comprehensively evaluate the robustness of the whole algorithm.

The experimental data mainly comes from the ISIC 2019 online public dataset. With the help of some dermatologists at the People's Liberation Army General Hospital of China, the dermatoscopic images with typical color anomalies are obtained, which cover various typical color deviation issues.

The experimental environments including the IBM computer in the experiments are equipped with an Intel Xeon (R) CPU E5-2678 v3 @ 2.50 GHz * 48 processor, 128 GB DDRAM, two NVDIA GeForce RTX 2080 Ti cards and the x64 bit Python with Linux.

### *2.3.1 The Image Fusion Experiment*

In this section, the gamma correction experimental results are presented in Fig. 2.5 for five dermoscopic images with the color and brightness constraints, including the uncorrected original image in Fig. 2.5a, the correction results with the unchanged color mean constraint in Fig. 2.5b, and the correction results under the unchanged brightness mean constraint in Fig. 2.5c. And further, the comparison results among the color correction methods based on the artificial fish swarms and other common color fusion algorithms are provided in Fig. 2.6. Due to the fact that the color correction carried out in this chapter mainly focuses on the low-frequency information of the image, some fixed fusion strategies for the high-frequency information such as the guided filtering method, the regional variance method, the weighted average method, the maximum value method, and the minimum value method, are adopted as the comparison algorithms to fuse the low-frequency part of the image. Here the radius of the guided filtering method is set with 4, and its regularization parameter is set with 0.1, and the weighting coefficient of the weighted average method is set with 0.5.

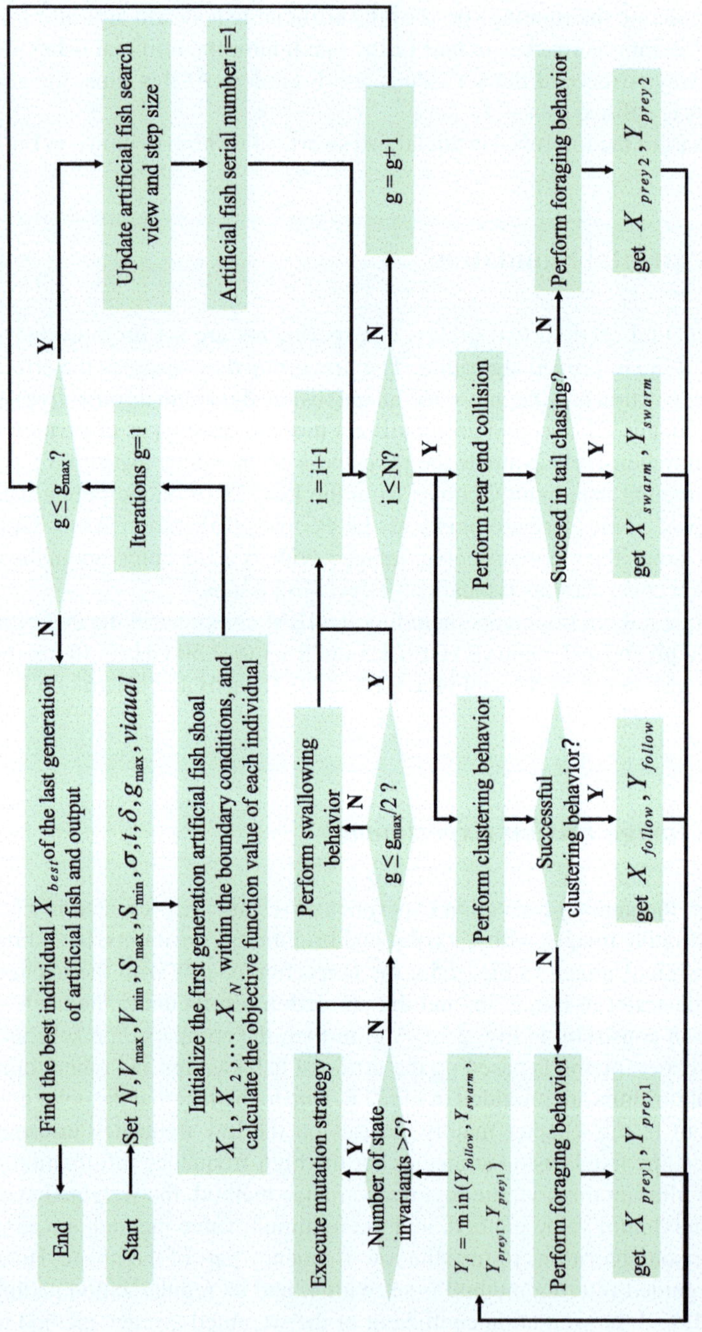


**Fig. 2.4** The improved artificial fish swarm algorithm

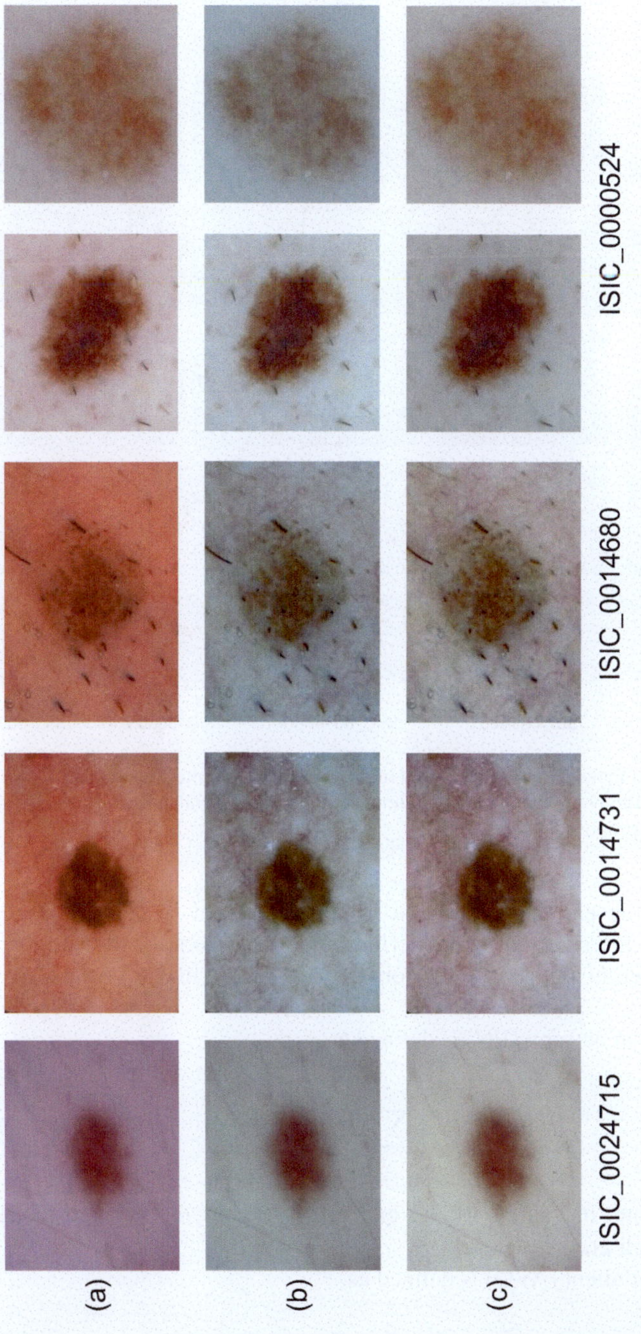


**Fig. 2.5** Color correction primary experiment results (**a** original image, **b** correction results under constant color mean constraint, **c** correction results under constant brightness mean constraint)

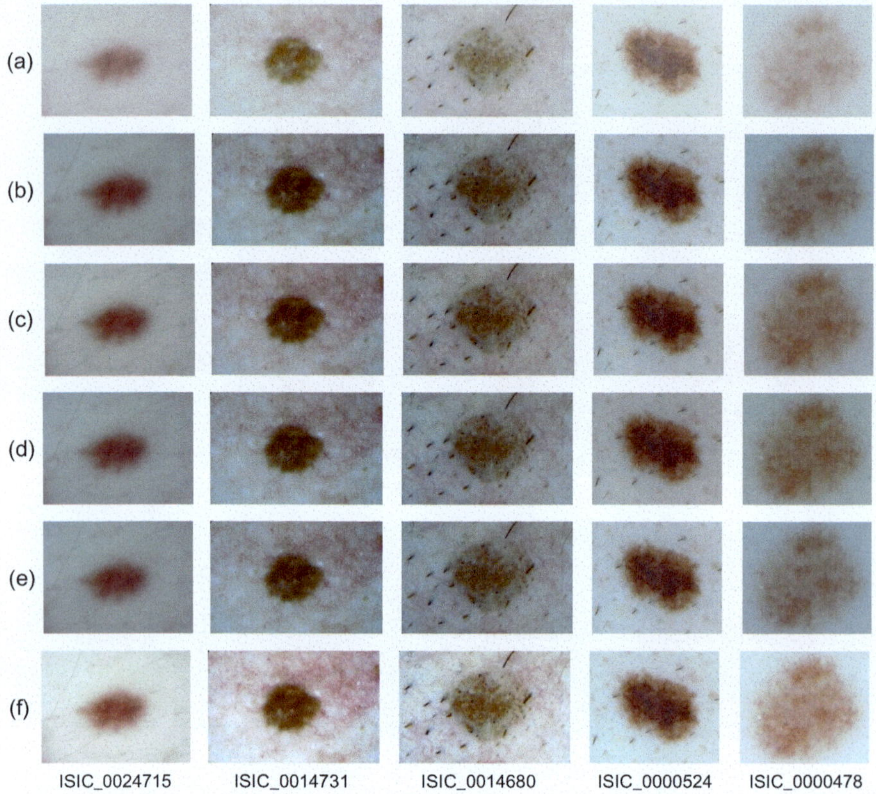


**Fig. 2.6** The experimental results of the fused image (**a** the guided filtering method, **b** the regional variance method, **c** the weighted average method, **d** the maximum value method, **e** the minimum value method, **f** the proposed algorithm)

The information entropy (2.28), the average gradient (2.29), and the spatial frequency (2.30) are selected as the performance indicators to evaluate the fusion results of the different algorithms, the corresponding experimental results are shown in Fig. 2.7.

The information entropy (EN) is defined as

$$EN = -\sum_{i=0}^{L-1} p_i \times \log_2 p_i \tag{2.28}$$

where $L$ represents the pixels of the entire image, and $p_i$ does the distribution probability of each grayscale level.

The average gradient (AVG) is defined as

$$AVG = \frac{1}{MN}\sum_{i=1}^{M}\sum_{j=1}^{N}\sqrt{\left(\Delta I_x^2 + \Delta I_y^2\right)\Big/ 2} \tag{2.29}$$

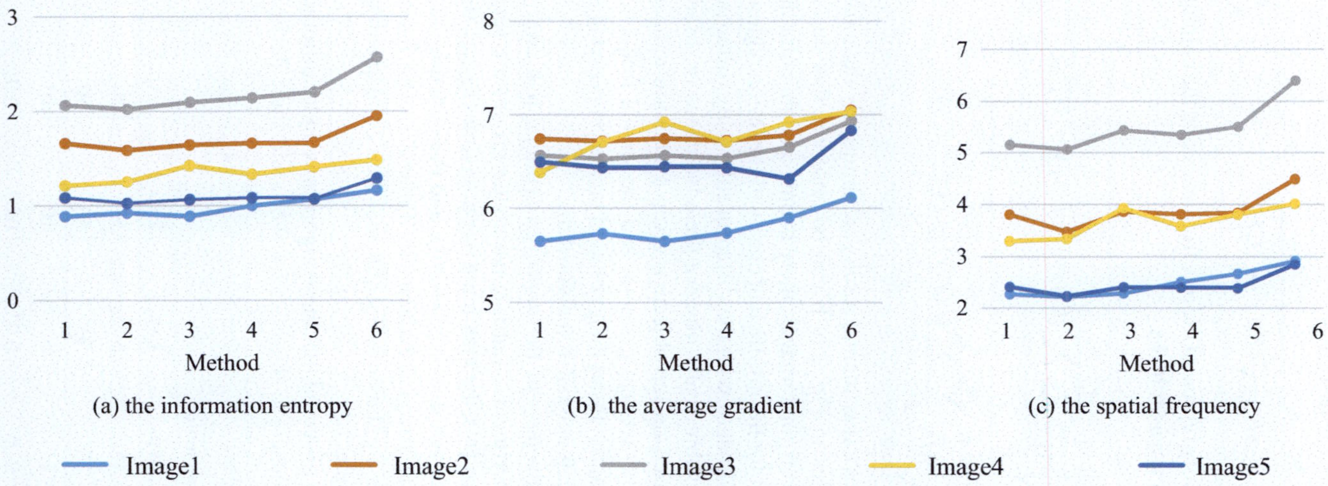


**Fig. 2.7** The experimental results of the different evaluation indexes (**a** the information entropy, **b** the average gradient, **c** the spatial frequency, method 1 denotes the guided filtering method, method 2 does the regional variance method; method 3 does weighted average method, method 4 does the maximum method, method 5 does the minimum method, method 6 does the proposed algorithm)

where $\Delta I_x = f(x, y) - f(x-1, y)$, $\Delta I_y = f(x, y) - f(x, y-1)$.

The spatial frequency (SF) is defined as

$$SF = \sqrt{(RF)^2 + (CF)^2} \tag{2.30}$$

where $RF$ and $CF$ respectively represent the row frequency and the column frequency, their calculation equations are as follows

$$RF = \sqrt{\frac{1}{MN}\sum_{x=1}^{M}\sum_{y=2}^{N}(f(x, y) - f(x, y-1))^2} \tag{2.31}$$

$$CF = \sqrt{\frac{1}{MN}\sum_{x=2}^{M}\sum_{y=1}^{N}(f(x, y) - f(x-1, y))^2} \tag{2.32}$$

The dermoscopic images experimental results are intuitively demonstrated based on the different fusion rules in Fig. 2.6. It can be observed that due to the small deviation between the two original images, there is only a slight color deviation and brightness deviation except for the insufficient clarity of the lesion region through the guided filtering, the fused images with the different rules only differ in brightness. However, it is difficult to subjectively observe the advantages or disadvantages of different fused results. Based on the objective given evaluation indicators such as the information entropy, the average gradient, and the spatial frequency, it can be observed and/or proved that the fused images based on the proposed algorithm have the optimal results among all comparison algorithms.

Furthermore, the effectiveness of the improved artificial fish swarm algorithm is verified. During the experiments, multiple parameter groups are set, such as the total of artificial fish swarms ($N$), the maximum iteration times ($g_{\max}$), the maximum probing times ($t$), the perceived distance ($visual$), and the crowding factor ($\delta$), and the selected different value arrays are shown in Table 2.1. The fusion results of different parameter settings are shown in Fig. 2.8, and their corresponding evaluation indicators are shown in Table 2.2.

From Fig. 2.8, it can be observed that these algorithms under different parameter settings can fuse the dermoscopic images very well, and their deviations are not

**Table 2.1** The parameter setting table

| Parameters | Exp. 1 | Exp. 2 | Exp. 3 | Exp. 4 | Exp. 5 | Exp. 6 |
|---|---|---|---|---|---|---|
| N | 15 | 15 | 5 | 5 | 20 | 20 |
| $g_{\max}$ | 20 | 30 | 50 | 50 | 50 | 50 |
| t | 5 | 5 | 5 | 10 | 10 | 10 |
| visual | 0.05 | 0.05 | 0.03 | 0.03 | 0.05 | 0.05 |
| $\delta$ | 0.139 | 0.139 | 0.139 | 0.139 | 0.139 | 0.3 |

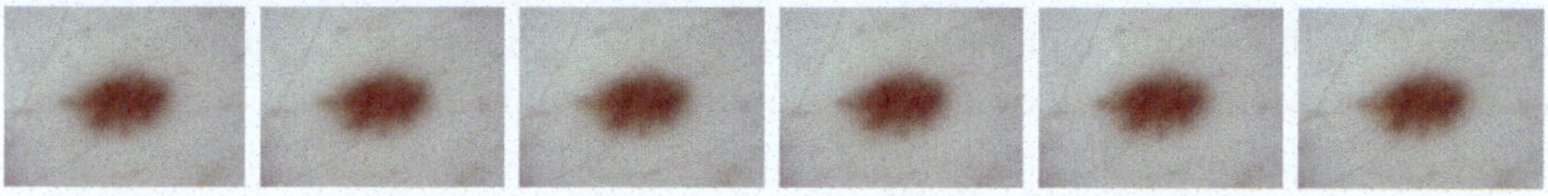


**Fig. 2.8** The fusion experiments of the dermoscopic images under different parameter settings (**a** Exp. 1, **b** Exp. 2, **c** Exp. 3, **d** Exp. 4, **e** Exp. 5, **f** Exp. 6)

**Table 2.2** The experimental evaluation index results

| Indicators | Exp. 1 | Exp. 2 | Exp. 3 | Exp. 4 | Exp. 5 | Exp. 6 |
|---|---|---|---|---|---|---|
| EN | 1.1407 | 1.1407 | 1.1508 | 1.1599 | 1.1513 | 1.1591 |
| AVG | 6.0998 | 6.1119 | 6.1391 | 6.1311 | 6.1232 | 6.1130 |
| SF | 2.9814 | 2.9937 | 2.9161 | 2.9268 | 2.9839 | 2.9141 |

significant. Through further analyzing the evaluation indicators in Table 2.2, it can be found that although there are some significant differences in the initial values and parameter settings for the designed six experiments, there is only a very small deviations in the results, and these deviations of the simulation diagrams are not been visually recognized. It demonstrates that the artificial fish swarm algorithm has a certain adaptive search ability, and does not be highly dependent on the initial values. That is to say that these randomly generating or setting initial values can reach to the fixed values. Therefore, it induces that the proposed algorithm does not highly depend on the parameter settings and holds a certain allowable range. In short, the proposed artificial fish swarm algorithm is not sensitive to the parameter settings and contributes to the stability of image fusion.

### 2.3.2 *The Comprehensive Color Correction Experiment*

In order to further validate the effectiveness and robustness of the overall proposed algorithms, their performances are provided in the following eight common skin diseases, such as the Actinic Keratosis (AK), the Basal Cell Carcinoma (BCC), the Benign Keratosis (BKL), the Dermatofibroma (DF), the Melanoma (MEL), the Nevus (NV), the Squamous cell carcinoma (SCC) and the vascular skin disease (VASC). Six typical dermatoscopy images are selected from each group of the experimental results, and the detailed comparative experimental results and the objective evaluation indicators are all provided.

The degree of color deviation correction in the images is measured by the evaluation indicators *Agva* and *Agvb*, which respectively represent the mean values of the channel *a* and the channel *b* in the Lab color space [16]. There are some modes in the Lab color space, i.e. the positive number of *a* represents "red", and its negative number represents "green"; while the positive number of *b* represents "yellow", and its corresponding negative number represents "blue". The larger the values of *Agva*, *Agvb* are, the more severe their color deviations are, while the smaller their absolute values are, the stronger the color correction ability of the model is. The degree of the features preservation of the lesion region after correction is achieved by extracting the lesion region from the image, and calculating the mean of the first and the second moment in the different color channels as the final evaluation indicator for the local features. The closer the indicator of the lesion region after correction is to the original image, the greater the preservation of the local features of the lesion during the correction process.

The performances of different color correction algorithms are shown in various skin diseases in Figs. 2.9, 2.10, 2.11, 2.12, 2.13, 2.14, 2.15 and 2.16. The comparative algorithms used in the above experiment include the shadow of grey (SOG), the image sharpening with gamma correction (ISGC), the gamma correction with constraints (GCC), the gamma correction, and the multi scale image fusion (GCMF). Here, the p-value in the Minkowski paradigm of the SOG algorithm is 6, and the gamma correction parameters in the ISGC and the GCC algorithms are the same as those in the GCMF. The objective evaluation indicators corresponding to the experimental results are listed after each group of images, whose part A provides the Avga/Avgb metrics for the images, whose part B does the first-order moment mean/second-order moment mean indicators for the lesion region. All optimal indicators in the tables are highlighted in bold font with underline. Finally, all indicators in the eight experimental results are statistically analyzed and presented in Figs. 2.17 and 2.18 (Tables 2.3, 2.4, 2.5, 2.6, 2.7, 2.8, 2.9, 2.10, 2.11, 2.12, 2.13, 2.14, 2.15, 2.16, 2.17, and 2.18).

Firstly, it can be intuitively observed from Figs. 2.9b, 2.10b, 2.11b, 2.12b, 2.13b, 2.14b, 2.15b and 2.16b that although the SOG method can deal with the color deviation in many cases, its ability to completely solve the color deviation in the images is restricted. For example, from Fig. 2.9b, it can be shown that there is the obvious deviation for the correction results for ISIC_ No. 0024511 and ISIC_No. 0024654 and it is invalid. From Figs. 2.13b and 2.14b, it can be obvious that there exists overall low brightness of the correction image and it is powerless to address the color tone deviation in the image. Then from Figs. 2.9c, 2.10c, 2.11c, 2.12c, 2.13c, 2.14c, 2.15c and 2.16c, it can be intuitively shown that the ISGC method poorly performs in terms of overall fusion results. In Figs. 2.13c and 2.14c, there exist even cases where the overall primary colors of the image significantly deviate from the reality. And then from Figs. 2.9d, 2.10d, 2.11d, 2.12d, 2.13d, 2.14d, 2.15d and 2.16d, it can be seen that the overall correction results of the GCC method are good, but for the ISIC_ No. 0024800 and ISIC_No. 0025373, there is a serious deviation between the color features of the lesion region and the actual situation, which deviates from the original intention of color correction, i.e. the color features of the image are restored as much as possible. Fourthly, from Figs. 2.9e, 2.10e, 2.11e, 2.12e, 2.13e, 2.14e, 2.15e and 2.16e, it is the fact that the improved algorithm performs well in the various skin disease images, without any issues such as over correction or the color feature loss of the lesion region. Based on the objective existed evaluation indicators, the proposed algorithm performs the best in the vast majority of experiments. Except

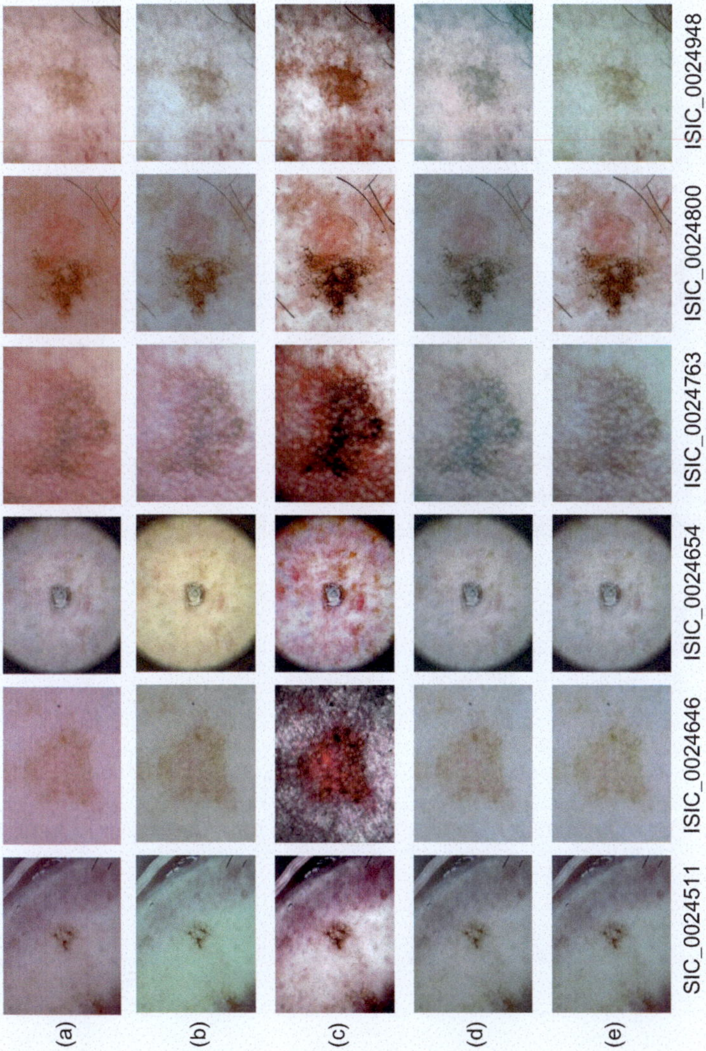


**Fig. 2.9** Results of color correction for the actinic keratosis (**a** the original images; **b** the SOG, **c** the ISGC, **d** the GCC, **e** the GCMF)

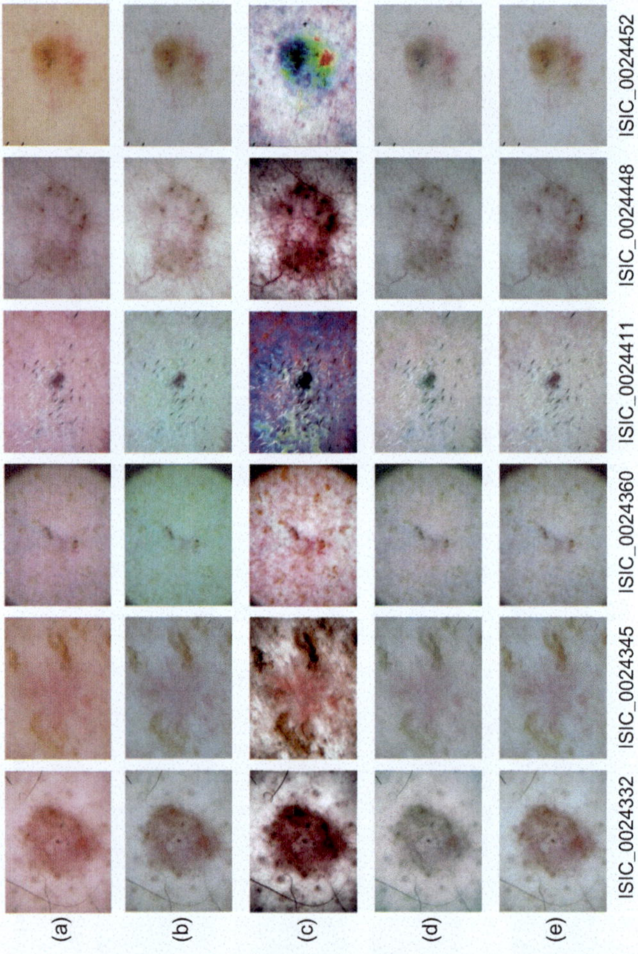


**Fig. 2.10** Color correction results for the basal cell carcinoma (**a** the original images; **b** the SOG, **c** the ISGC, **d** the GCC, **e** the GCMF)

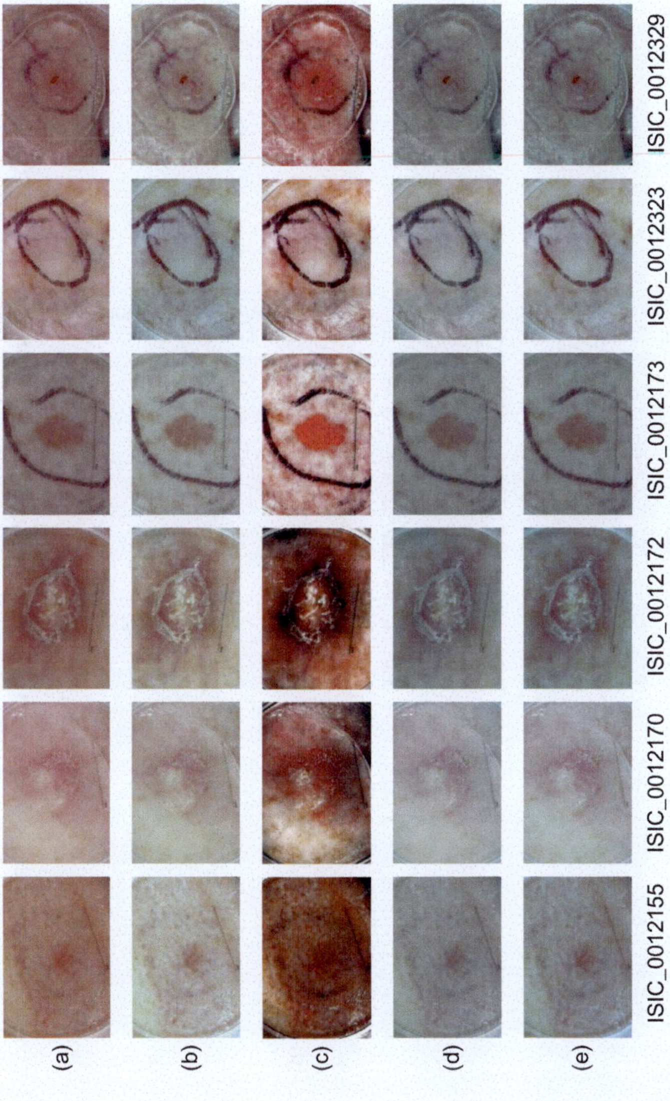


**Fig. 2.11** Results of color correction for the keratosis alba (**a** the original images; **b** the SOG, **c** the ISGC, **d** the GCC, **e** the GCMF)

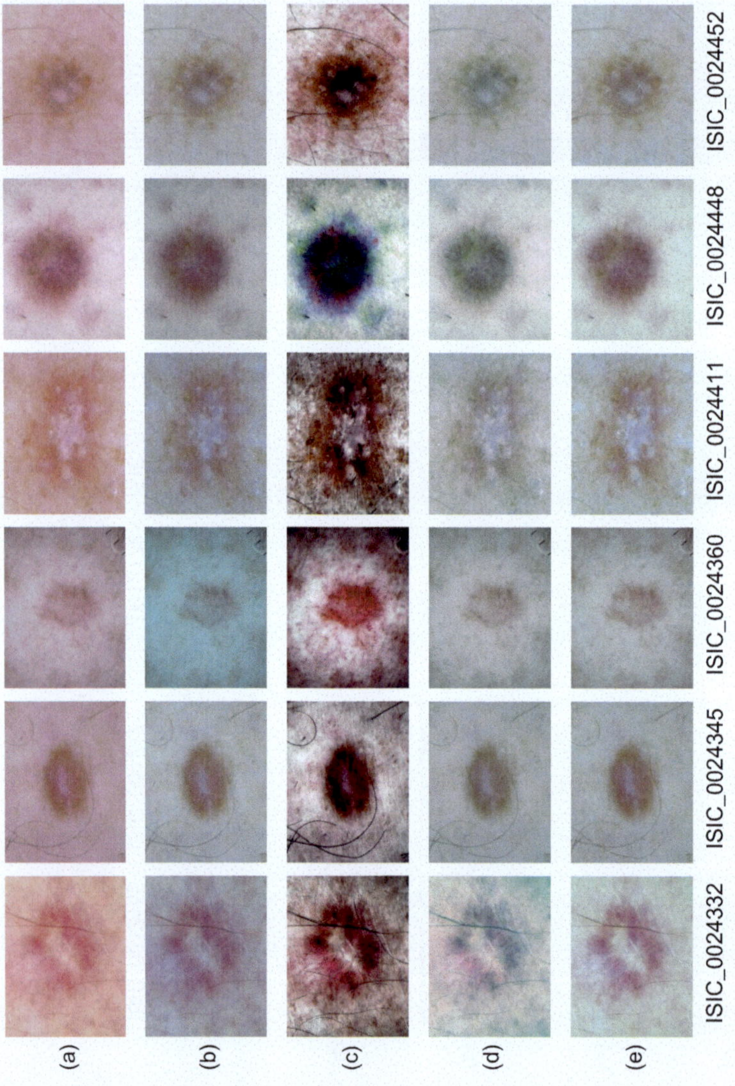


**Fig. 2.12** Results of color correction for the dermatofibromas (**a** the original images, **b** the SOG, **c** the ISGC, **d** the GCC, **e** the GCMF)

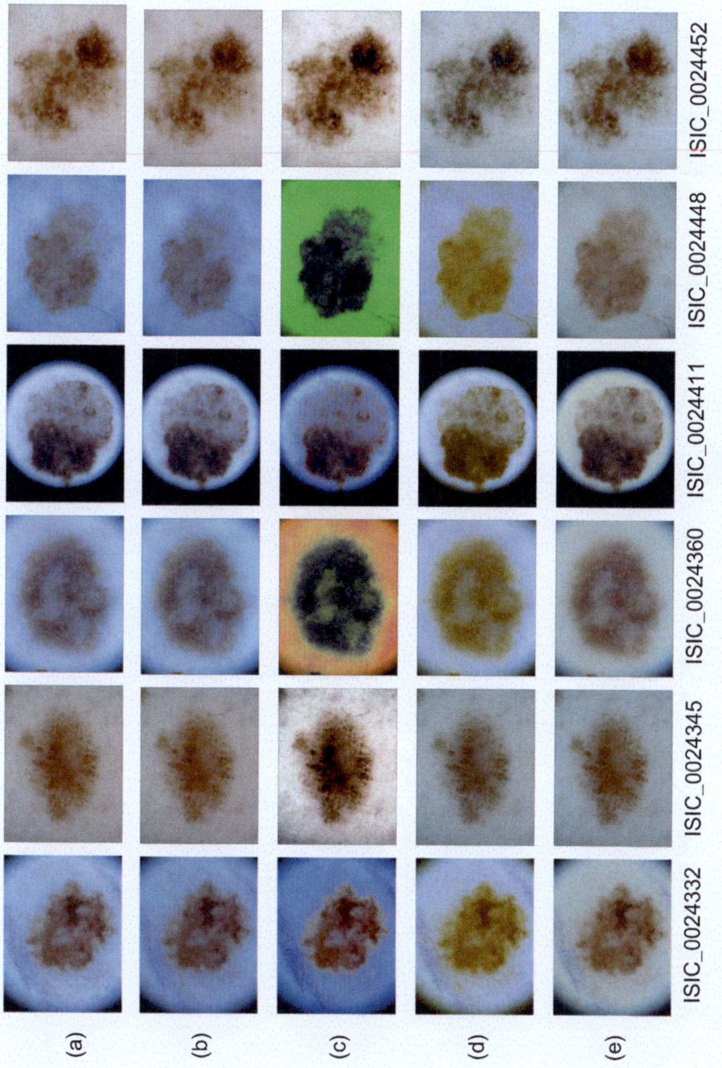


**Fig. 2.13** Color correction results for the melanoma (**a** the original image; **b** the SOG, **c** the ISGC, **d** the GCC, **e** the GCMF)

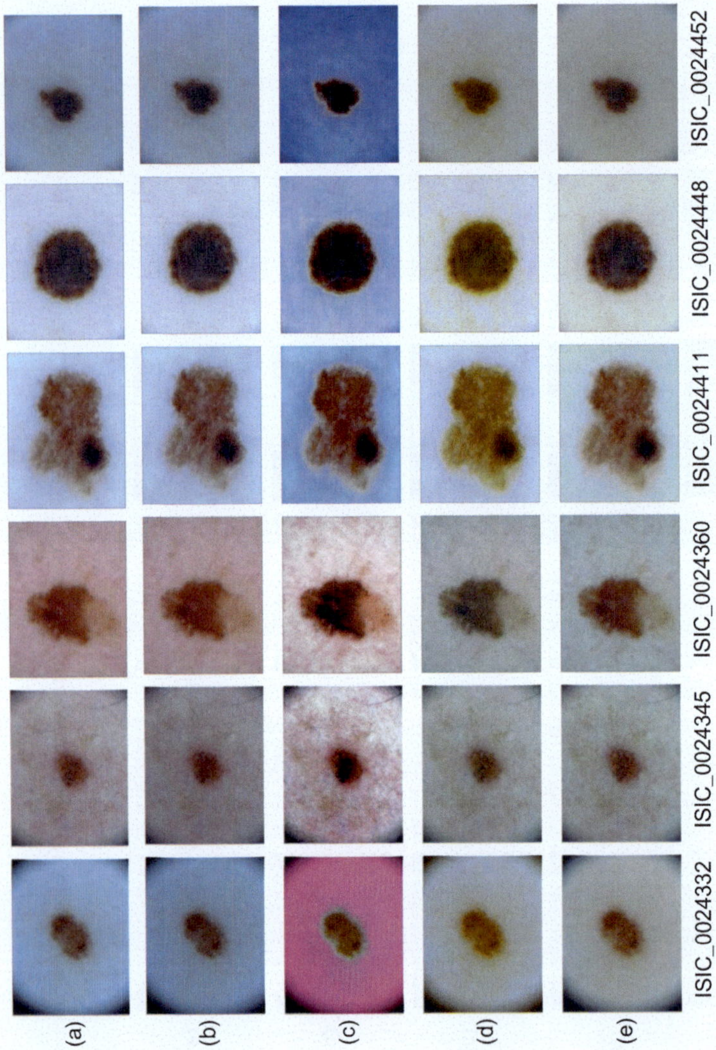


**Fig. 2.14** Results of color correction experiments for the melanocytic nevi (**a** the original image; **b** the SOG, **c** the ISGC, **d** the GCC, **e** the GCMF)

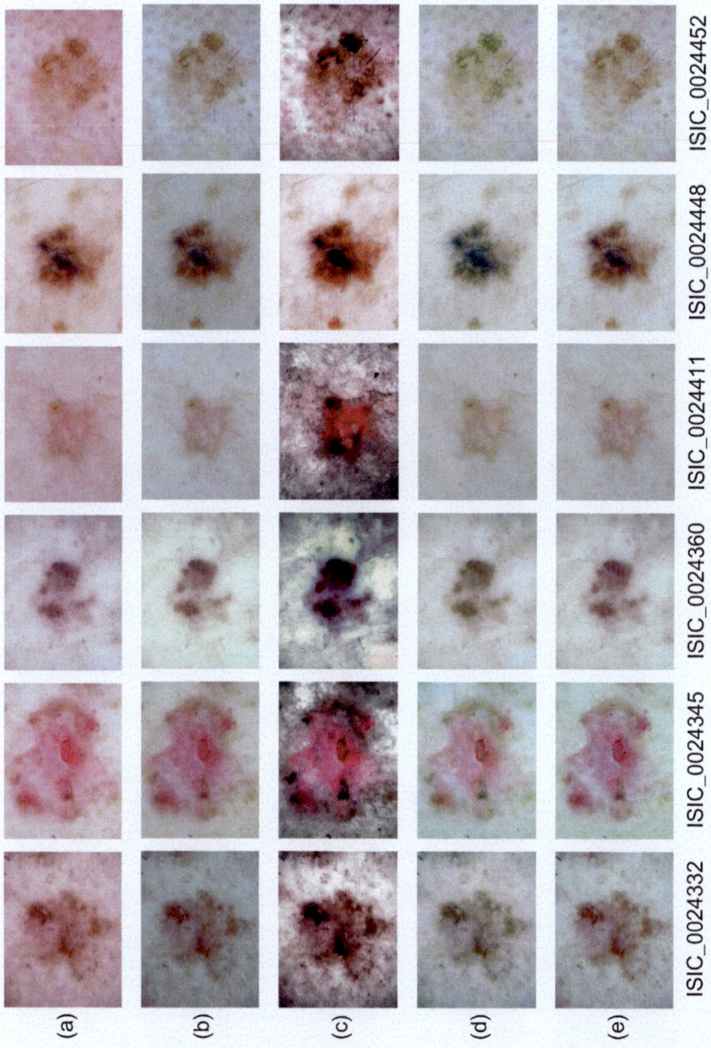


**Fig. 2.15** Color correction results for the squamous cell carcinoma (**a** the original image; **b** the SOG, **c** the ISGC, **d** the GCC, **e** the GCMF)

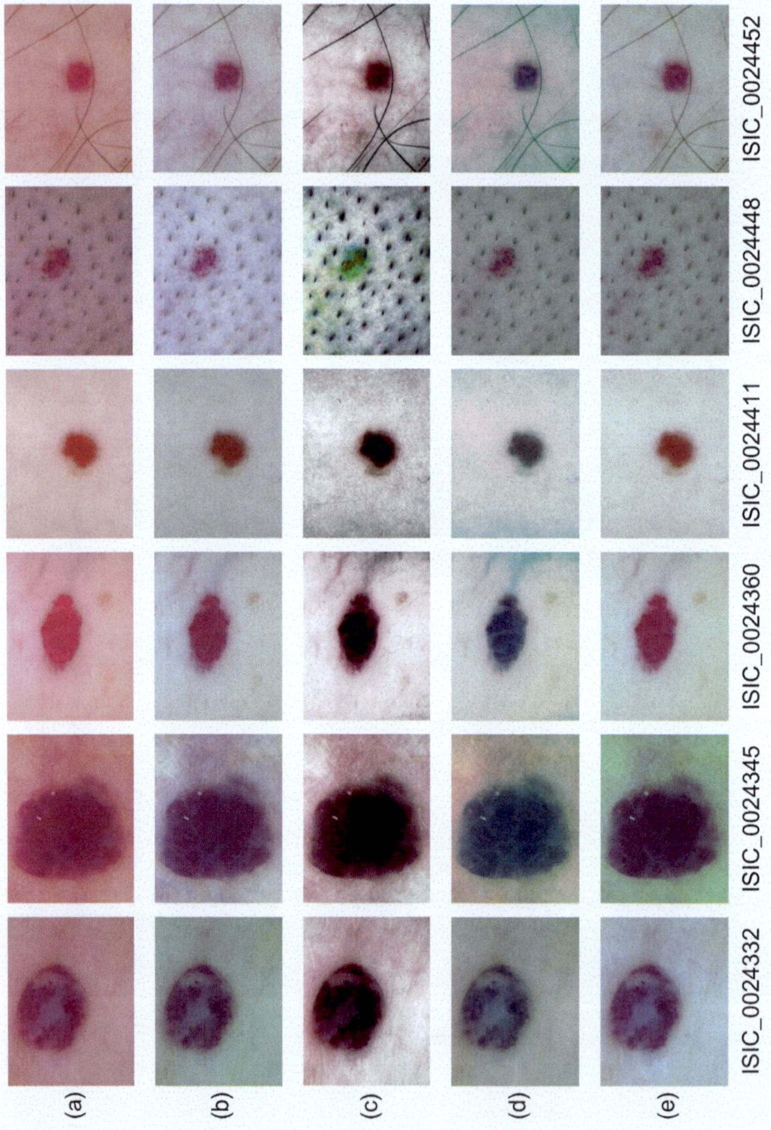


**Fig. 2.16** Color correction results for the vascular skin diseases (**a** the original images; **b** the SOG, **c** the ISGC, **d** the GCC, **e** the GCMF)

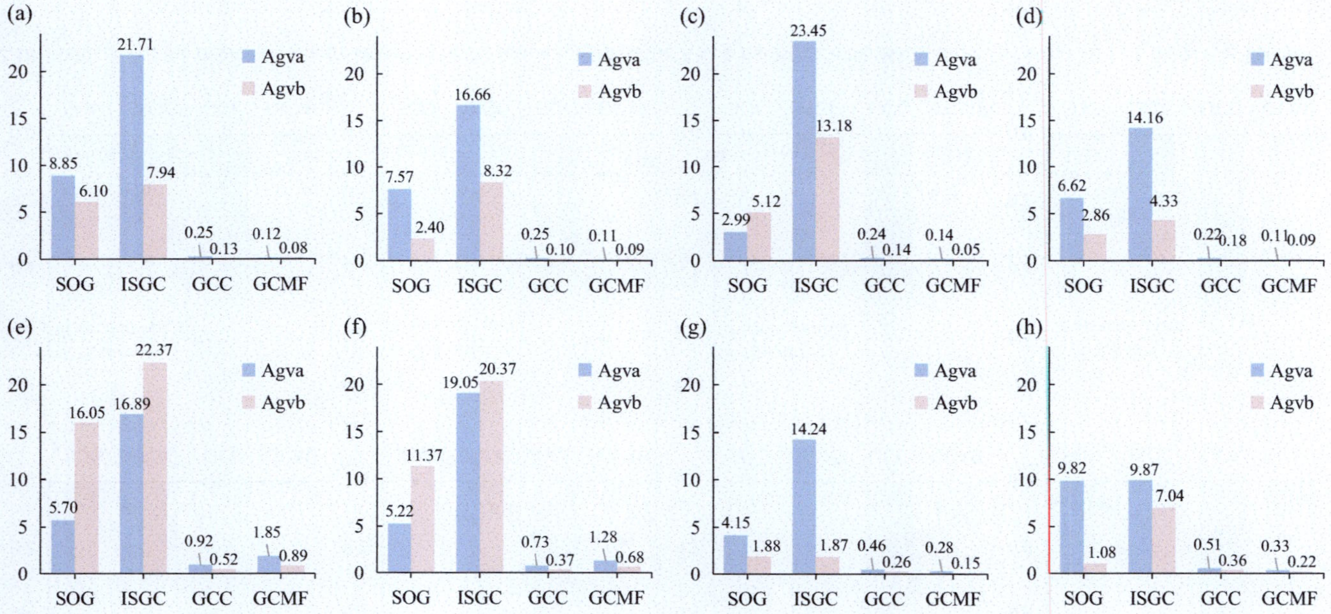


**Fig. 2.17** Chromatic aberration correction statistics for color correction (**a** the AK, **b** the BCC, **c** the BKL, **d** the DF, **e** the MEL, **f** the NV, **g** the SCC, **h** the VASC)

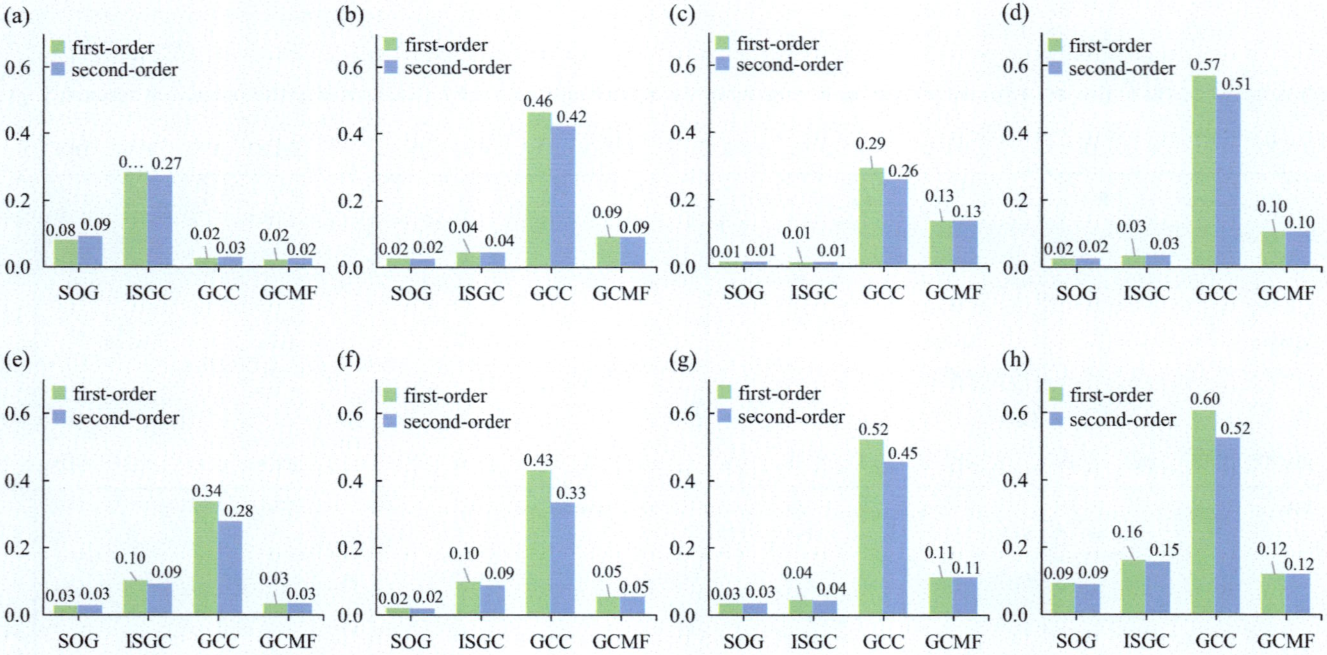


**Fig. 2.18** Statistics of the degree of feature retention in the lesion region (**a** the AK, **b** the BCC, **c** the BKL, **d** the DF, **e** the MEL, **f** the NV, **g** The SCC, **h** the VASC)

**Table 2.3** Results of color correction for the actinic keratosis (chromatic aberration correction)

| | Original image | SOG | ISGC | GCC | GCMF |
|---|---|---|---|---|---|
| ISIC_ 0024511 | 16.375/– 4.312 | – 14.013/– 3.738 | 19.676/ 6.514 | 0.32/0.062 | **0.188/0.042** |
| ISIC_ 0024646 | 21.027/– 4.288 | 1.514/– 0.098 | 21.781/ 6.041 | **0.159**/0.145 | 0.238/**0.081** |
| ISIC_ 0024654 | 8.174/– 1.339 | 2.52/– 0.228 | 20.466/ 21.897 | 0.091/**– 0.005** | **– 0.09**/0.08 |
| ISIC_ 0024763 | 29.156/ 9.954 | 18.007/13.43 | 31.115/– 1.862 | 0.27/0.174 | **0.007/– 0.046** |
| ISIC_ 0024800 | 27.449/ 14.384 | 6.276/10.777 | 19.739/ 3.112 | 0.468/0.278 | **0.152/0.131** |
| ISIC_ 0024948 | 19.022/ 7.397 | – 10.76/8.328 | 17.488/ 8.243 | 0.198/**0.112** | **0.059**/0.129 |

**Table 2.4** Results of color correction for the actinic keratosis (the degree of lesion regional feature preservation)

| | Original image | SOG | ISGC | GCC | GCMF |
|---|---|---|---|---|---|
| ISIC_ 0024511 | 40.554/ 68.98 | 46.011/78.308 | 48.876/85.183 | 39.164/66.636 | **39.338/66.941** |
| ISIC_ 0024646 | 53.599/ 79.537 | 48.08/71.344 | 31.246/53.786 | 51.523/76.462 | **51.66/76.67** |
| ISIC_ 0024654 | 17.083/ 52.517 | 19.2/58.99 | 18.12757.113 | 16.828/51.717 | **16.885/51.913** |
| ISIC_ 0024763 | 5.062/ 26.535 | 5.66/29.672 | 2.288/13.391 | **4.924/25.822** | 2.853/14.464 |
| ISIC_ 0024800 | 6.747/ 29.098 | 6.808/29.389 | 7.644/34.046 | 6.535/28.219 | **6.731/29.037** |
| ISIC_ 0024948 | 3.337/ 23.254 | 3.156/22.001 | 2.108/15.859 | 3.276/22.84 | **3.277/22.849** |

with the basal cell carcinoma and the melanoma images, the objective evaluation of the GCC method is better. Although the ISGC method has the best experimental results in several individual experiments, due to its poor subjective effect and small proportion, it does not have universal sense. Finally, analyzing the comprehensive performance of the experiments, it can be seen from Fig. 2.17 that based on the average value of evaluation indicators, the GCC method has the best color deviation correction effect in the images, while the ISGC method performs the worst. Although the proposed algorithm is slightly inferior to the GCC method in some images, its overall performance is stable and the gap with the GCC method is very small. Based on Fig. 2.18, although the GCC method has the best color deviation

**Table 2.5** Color correction results for the basal cell carcinoma (chromatic aberration correction)

| | Original image | SOG | ISGC | GCC | GCMF |
|---|---|---|---|---|---|
| ISIC_0024332 | 21.452/ 3.739 | 2.266/1.503 | 13.249/ 3.414 | 0.373/0.276 | **0.054/0.137** |
| ISIC_0024345 | 19.360/ 10.57 | 1.868/– 0.056 | 18.115/ 9.981 | 0.197/0.045 | **0.115/0.031** |
| ISIC_0024360 | 14.298/– 0.39 | – 20.274/ 6.461 | 19.522/ 1.601 | 0.13/**0.14** | **– 0.07**/0.163 |
| ISIC_0024411 | 22.703/ 5.114 | – 14.151/ 1.892 | 25.024/– 26.491 | 0.221/**0.009** | **0.059**/0.082 |
| ISIC_0024448 | 14.524/ 0.63 | 4.262/2.856 | 19.896/ 1.567 | 0.201/**– 0.04** | **0.184**/– 0.115 |
| ISIC_0024452 | 11.674/ 18.204 | 2.577/1.655 | 4.151/– 6.886 | 0.387/0.104 | **0.177/0.004** |

**Table 2.6** Color correction results for the basal cell carcinoma (the degree of lesion regional feature preservation)

| | Original image | SOG | ISGC | GCC | GCMF |
|---|---|---|---|---|---|
| ISIC_ 0024332 | 37.695/ 65.25 | 33.31/57.693 | 16.838/32.901 | 36.435/63.114 | **36.479/63.168** |
| ISIC_ 0024345 | 68.628/ 81.364 | 64.472/76.46 | 69.282/84.264 | 68.396/**81.113** | **68.41**/81.057 |
| ISIC_ 0024360 | 1.23/ 13.58 | 1.184/13.086 | 1.101/12.579 | 1.2/13.262 | **1.207/13.325** |
| ISIC_ 0024411 | 0.459/ 6.825 | **0.442**/6.57 | 0.005/0.213 | 0.435/**6.468** | 0.39/5.813 |
| ISIC_ 0024448 | 53.799/ 68.957 | 65.172/83.548 | 31.891/45.796 | **52.526/67.347** | 52.446/67.217 |
| ISIC_ 0024452 | 3.335/ 19.616 | 3.075/18.098 | 0.975/7.601 | **3.294/19.387** | 3.444/20.272 |

**Table 2.7** Results of color correction for the keratosis alba (chromatic aberration correction)

| | Original image | SOG | ISGC | GCC | GCMF |
|---|---|---|---|---|---|
| ISIC_0012155 | 18.436/14.627 | – 1.291/6.832 | 24.060/19.845 | 0.161/0.163 | **0.103/0.04** |
| ISIC_0012170 | 13.572/7.631 | 2.112/7.107 | 20.666/13.538 | 0.181/0.104 | **0.108/0.011** |
| ISIC_0012172 | 20.013/10.611 | 7.025/9.121 | 25.830/16.307 | 0.308/0.163 | **0.130/0.067** |
| ISIC_0012173 | 11.458/3.7 | 0.174/2.829 | 22.091/9.650 | 0.14/**0.114** | **0.121**/0.125 |
| ISIC_0012323 | 15.751/6.836 | – 1.126/0.253 | 16.661/8.357 | 0.397/0.162 | **0.238/– 0.012** |
| ISIC_0012329 | 22.077/6.085 | 6.216/4.555 | 31.417/11.359 | 0.232/0.123 | **0.165/0.02** |

**Table 2.8** Results of color correction for the keratosis alba (the degree of lesion regional feature preservation)

| | Original image | SOG | ISGC | GCC | GCMF |
|---|---|---|---|---|---|
| ISIC_0012155 | 29.266/56.056 | 13.829/28.045 | 36.211/69.393 | 29.5/56.46 | **29.277/56.112** |
| ISIC_0012170 | 98.96/82.965 | 61.883/59.992 | 98.357/82.472 | 98.552/82.648 | **98.856/82.786** |
| ISIC_0012172 | 20.887/44.027 | 6.784/18.533 | 24.985/52.69 | 20.505/43.281 | **20.669/43.492** |
| ISIC_0012173 | 8.326/30.687 | 8.164/32.594 | 9.786/36.083 | 8.181/30.166 | **8.247/30.385** |
| ISIC_0012323 | 49.183/75.876 | 51.646/80.57 | 47.848/73.843 | 48.856/75.323 | **48.908/75.475** |
| ISIC_0012329 | 38.855/57.278 | 35.115/54.032 | 44.997/66.39 | 37.754/55.726 | **37.872/55.813** |

**Table 2.9** Results of color correction for the dermatofibromas (chromatic aberration correction)

| | Original image | SOG | ISGC | GCC | GCMF |
|---|---|---|---|---|---|
| ISIC_0024553 | 27.498/9.432 | 11.552/−6.366 | 18.730/6.665 | 0.278/0.122 | **0.126/0.072** |
| ISIC_0024845 | 16.109/1.235 | 1.518/−0.953 | 11.446/1.621 | 0.277/0.184 | **0.229/0.05** |
| ISIC_0025154 | 12.346/−0.756 | − 9.672/−5.632 | 19.842/1.638 | **0.031**/0.193 | 0.067/**0.105** |
| ISIC_0025223 | 21.476/8.623 | 6.561/−2.491 | 15.704/7.216 | 0.261/0.179 | **0.137/0.069** |
| ISIC_0025373 | 18.461/−1.757 | 6.223/−0.996 | − 0.908/−3.217 | 0.292/0.265 | **− 0.044/0.18** |
| ISIC_0025668 | 19.355/4.016 | 4.179/0.711 | 18.347/5.637 | 0.202/0.125 | **0.039/0.051** |

correction effect, it alters the color characteristics of the lesion region to a large extent. On the basis of realizing the color correction task, the optimization algorithm preserves the color features of the lesion region to the greatest extent. For overall performances, the proposed algorithm is the optimal. Due to the different challenges present in different skin disease images, for example the common drawback in the melanoma and the nevus images is the deviation of brightness and color tone, the more common imperfection in the actinic keratosis and the basal cell carcinoma is the overall image redness. For different skin diseases, except for the proposed algorithm performs stably, other algorithms exhibit significant flaws in performance across different types of images.

**Table 2.10** Results of color correction for the dermatofibromas (the degree of lesion regional feature preservation)

| | Original image | SOG | ISGC | GCC | GCMF |
|---|---|---|---|---|---|
| ISIC_0024553 | 1.916/19.895 | 1.63/16.93 | 1.829/19.162 | 1.965/20.408 | **1.887/19.605** |
| ISIC_0024845 | 17.34/45.453 | **17.388/45.589** | 4.581/14.96 | 16.825/44.114 | 16.873/44.207 |
| ISIC_0025154 | 8.792/36.162 | 7.913/32.556 | 4.788/21.411 | 8.592/35.342 | **8.655/35.595** |
| ISIC_0025223 | 69.167/82.659 | 61.004/72.94 | 28.443/40.204 | 68.069/81.396 | **68.335/81.508** |
| ISIC_0025373 | 19.238/47.34 | 15.512/38.175 | 3.633/11.613 | 17.682/43.55 | **18.519/45.582** |
| ISIC_0025668 | 14.343/43.604 | 13.519/41.099 | 3.369/13.785 | 13.833/42.033 | **13.977/42.491** |

**Table 2.11** Color correction results for the melanoma (chromatic aberration correction)

| | Original image | SOG | ISGC | GCC | GCMF |
|---|---|---|---|---|---|
| ISIC_0000002 | 4.530/– 19.766 | 5.166/– 18.599 | 12.405/– 32.475 | **1.085/0.744** | 2.880/1.314 |
| ISIC_0000022 | 7.443/5.812 | 7.415/5.741 | 8.377/6.232 | 0.935/0.514 | **0.704/0.366** |
| ISIC_0000035 | 4.392/– 20.386 | 2.292/– 18.124 | 11.366/21.225 | **0.865/0.324** | 2.517/1.401 |
| ISIC_0000036 | 3.540/– 12.822 | 3.514/– 12.652 | 8.687/– 19.82 | **0.773/0.185** | 1.494/0.913 |
| ISIC_0000046 | 3.567/– 25.88 | 6.061/– 32.303 | – 50.035/44.891 | **0.653/0.381** | 3.008/0.903 |
| ISIC_0000049 | 10.017/8.34 | 9.754/8.857 | 10.479/9.597 | 1.234/0.945 | **0.526/0.445** |

**Table 2.12** Color correction results for the melanoma (the degree of lesion regional feature preservation)

| | Original image | SOG | ISGC | GCC | GCMF |
|---|---|---|---|---|---|
| ISIC_0000002 | 20.895/42.146 | 18.28/36.87 | 17.517/36.487 | **20.564/41.412** | 17.735/36.043 |
| ISIC_0000022 | 22.809/42.652 | 22.497/42.056 | 16.872/35.684 | 22.505/42.168 | **22.885/42.746** |
| ISIC_0000035 | 42.453/58.179 | **41.358/56.684** | 19.783/31.085 | 40.898/55.99 | 36.695/50.845 |
| ISIC_0000036 | 9.496/24.791 | **9.364/24.451** | 8.762/23.028 | 9.178/23.956 | 8.042/21.148 |
| ISIC_0000046 | 20.404/46.301 | **20.605/46.792** | 5.448/17.007 | 19.69/44.555 | 17.078/40.565 |
| ISIC_0000049 | 12.446/30.913 | 12.315/30.591 | 9.225/25.048 | 12.147/30.252 | **12.436/30.947** |

**Table 2.13** Results of color correction experiments for the melanocytic nevi (chromatic aberration correction)

| | Original image | SOG | ISGC | GCC | GCMF |
|---|---|---|---|---|---|
| ISIC_0000007 | – 1.163/– 18.155 | – 0.279/– 17.621 | 55.436/– 18.514 | 0.994/0.464 | **0.453/0.181** |
| ISIC_0000012 | 8.285/– 2.377 | 7.644/– 2.539 | 11.957/– 2.569 | **0.17**/0.179 | 0.212/**0.135** |
| ISIC_0000020 | 15.998/5.121 | 15.812/5.756 | 13.554/5.259 | **0.380/0.219** | 0.833/0.503 |
| ISIC_0000038 | 3.590/– 11.032 | 3.936/– 12.265 | 7.569/– 18.005 | 3.604/1.865 | **1.736/1.067** |
| ISIC_0000039 | 1.935/– 13.092 | 1.622/– 12.753 | 5.811/– 23.738 | 1.974/1.129 | **0.792/0.279** |
| ISIC_0000039 | 1.241/– 17.962 | 2.034/– 17.260 | 20.004/– 54.138 | 0.552/0.213 | **0.35/– 0.032** |

**Table 2.14** Results of color correction experiments for the melanocytic nevi (the degree of lesion regional feature preservation)

| | Original image | SOG | ISGC | GCC | GCMF |
|---|---|---|---|---|---|
| ISIC_0000007 | 6.693/23.88 | 5.834/20.823 | 6.005/22.636 | 6.068/21.829 | **6.719/23.894** |
| ISIC_0000012 | 1.892/11.327 | 1.639/9.809 | 0.56/4.256 | 1.802/10.809 | **1.842/11.028** |
| ISIC_0000020 | 16.198/36.855 | **15.85/36.048** | 10.807/30.82 | 15.579/35.615 | 15.567/35.548 |
| ISIC_0000038 | 44.412/59.828 | **44.144/59.493** | 34.5/51.809 | 43.698/58.663 | 39.492/55.335 |
| ISIC_0000039 | 10.137/23.268 | 10.325/23.668 | 4.231/11.73 | 8.269/19.205 | 10.004/22.963 |
| ISIC_0000039 | 2.722/12.406 | 2.674/12.189 | 1.007/5.78 | 2.41/11.017 | **2.676/12.2** |

**Table 2.15** Color correction results for the squamous cell carcinoma (chromatic aberration correction)

| | Original image | SOG | ISGC | GCC | GCMF |
|---|---|---|---|---|---|
| ISIC_0024372 | 20.225/1.219 | 2.706/− 0.265 | 13.796/1.742 | 0.539/0.289 | **0.273/0.085** |
| ISIC_0024710 | 24.243/− 2.607 | 12.480/1.76 | 20.404/− 0.429 | 0.661/0.625 | **0.536/0.48** |
| ISIC_0024925 | 10.034/− 6.028 | − 1.624/2.16 | 1.872/− 0.688 | 0.313/**0.051** | **0.292**/0.119 |
| ISIC_0024946 | 14.36/− 1.371 | 1.784/− 3.384 | 16.712/1.161 | **0.197**/0.044 | 0.241/**0.022** |
| ISIC_0025069 | 15.083/4.08 | 3.637/0.717 | 15.255/6.171 | 0.632/0.416 | **0.118/0.083** |
| ISIC_0025089 | 22.132/− 1.295 | 2.663/2.973 | 17.417/1.008 | 0.423/0.16 | **0.222/0.135** |

**Table 2.16** Color correction results for the squamous cell carcinoma (the degree of lesion regional feature preservation)

| | Original image | SOG | ISGC | GCC | GCMF |
|---|---|---|---|---|---|
| ISIC_0024372 | 18.046/45.559 | 14.405/36.408 | 9.415/26.501 | 17.283/43.691 | **17.313/43.767** |
| ISIC_0024710 | 77.288/94.891 | 67.01/82.341 | 60.996/78.843 | 74.094/91.181 | **75.489/92.364** |
| ISIC_0024925 | 14.755/43.699 | 15.33/45.422 | 5.549/20.297 | 14.373/**42.579** | **13.984**/41.537 |
| ISIC_0024946 | 1.415/14.463 | 1.389/14.207 | 0.247/3.185 | 1.378/14.089 | **1.38/14.115** |
| ISIC_0025069 | 7.797/26.7 | 6.24/21.349 | 4.112/16.269 | 7.204/24.877 | **7.55/25.841** |
| ISIC_0025089 | 20.15/51.641 | 18.573/47.619 | 9.88/29.143 | 19.212/49.314 | **19.345/49.598** |

**Table 2.17** Color correction results for the vascular skin diseases (chromatic aberration correction)

| | Original image | SOG | ISGC | GCC | GCMF |
|---|---|---|---|---|---|
| ISIC_0024370 | 31.726/1.365 | 6.431/0.413 | 14.382/− 10.008 | 0.745/**0.09** | **0.517**/− 0.317 |
| ISIC_0024662 | 46.038/3.753 | 23.839/0.742 | 17.618/− 11.748 | 1.384/**0.493** | **0.987**/− 0.601 |
| ISIC_0024706 | 30.411/3.681 | 6.636/0.677 | 8.794/− 2.604 | 0.243/0.942 | **0.215/− 0.182** |
| ISIC_0025197 | 17.654/6.13 | 2.431/1.414 | 3.909/0.82 | 0.485/0.328 | **0.022/0.034** |
| ISIC_0025250 | 24.861/− 0.033 | 10.174/1.696 | − 5.223/− 13.59 | 0.118/0.107 | **0.087/0.052** |
| ISIC_0025425 | 32.914/7.543 | 9.403/1.539 | 9.280/− 3.444 | **0.091**/0.184 | 0.169/**0.146** |

**Table 2.18** Color correction results for the vascular skin diseases (the degree of lesion regional feature preservation)

| | Original image | SOG | ISGC | GCC | GCMF |
|---|---|---|---|---|---|
| ISIC_0024370 | 29.423/50.978 | 32.161/55.963 | 15.823/34.6 | 26.546/46.192 | **27.163/47.322** |
| ISIC_0024662 | 28.161/42.506 | **28.047/42.495** | 8.154/15.942 | 21.003/32.133 | 23.741/36.149 |
| ISIC_0024706 | 11.442/35.646 | 10.108/31.644 | 3.326/13.957 | 8.628/27.272 | 10.286/32.249 |
| ISIC_0025197 | 3.647/19.268 | 3.038/16.075 | 0.411/3.158 | 3.117/16.499 | **3.444/18.226** |
| ISIC_0025250 | 6.364/27.771 | 8.271/36.183 | 5.179/24.957 | 5.994/26.251 | **6.038/26.343** |
| ISIC_0025425 | 2.238/15.591 | **2.154/15.025** | 0.732/5.572 | 1.875/13.093 | 2.007/14.008 |

## 2.4 Conclusion

A dermoscopic color correction algorithm is proposed based on the Newton iteration method for the gamma correction and the multi-scale image fusion, which conquers the color deviation in the dermoscopic images. Firstly, the color deviation criterion is formed as the objective function for the gamma correction. Through some classical stages such as smooth optimization of the objective function and Lagrangian duality, the constrained objective function is transformed into an unconstrained convex optimization problem. Then, the objective function is analytically soluble using the Newton iteration method, and the initial value dependency problem in the Newton iteration method is overcome using the binary method. For the multi-scale image fusion algorithm, a fusion method based on the regional energy is used for the high-frequency images after wavelet decomposition, and an optimized fusion method based on the artificial fish swarm algorithm is used for the low-frequency images to preserve the significant features of the original corrected image in different frequency domains as much as possible. The experiments demonstrate that the proposed algorithms can deal with the color correction with different constraints, which can achieve color correction of the image while preserving the color features of the lesion region as much as possible. The proposed algorithm is not sensitive to parameter settings, and ensures the stability of the experimental results, on the contrary, other existed algorithms exhibit significant flaws in performance across different types of skin disease images.

## References

1. Lee DJ, Faries MB. Practical manual for dermatologic and surgical melanoma management. Switzerland: Springer; 2021.
2. Javed R, Rahim MSM, Saba T, et al. A comparative study of features selection for skin lesion detection from dermoscopic images. Netw Modeli Anal Health Inform Bioinform. 2020;9:1–13.
3. Ezenwa E, Stein JA, Krueger L. Dermoscopic features of neoplasms in skin of color: A1 review. Int J Women's Dermatol. 2021;7(2):145–51.

4. Gutierrez D, Gaulding JV, Motta Beltran A, et al. Photodermatoses in skin of colour. J Eur Acad Dermatol Venereol. 2018;32(11):1879–86.
5. Lallas A, Reggiani C, Argenziano G, et al. Dermoscopic nevus patterns in skin of colour: a prospective, cross-sectional, morphological study in individuals with skin type V and VI. J Eur Acad Dermatol Venereol. 2014;28(11):1469–74.
6. Land EH, Mccann JJ. Lightness and retinex theory. Josa. 1971;61(1):1–11.
7. Land EH. Recent advances in retinex theory and some implications for cortical computations: color vision and the natural image. Proc Natl Acad Sci. 1983;80(16):5163–9.
8. Jang D-W, Park R-H. Color fringe correction by the color difference prediction using the logistic function. IEEE Trans Image Process. 2017;26(5):2561–70.
9. Sathish S, Sumithra MG, Mohanasundaram K. Shading and texture constrained retinex for correcting vignetting on dermatological macro images. Vis Comput. 2023;39(2):693–709.
10. Liang Z, Ding X, Jin J, et al. A color cast image enhancement method based on affine transform in poor visible conditions. IEEE Geosci Remote Sens Lett. 2022;19:1–5.
11. Ma J, Fan X, Yang SX, et al. Contrast limited adaptive histogram equalization-based fusion in YIQ and HSI color spaces for underwater image enhancement. Int J Pattern Recognit Artif Intell. 2018;32(07):1854018.
12. Tian Q-C, Cohen LD. A variational-based fusion model for non-uniform illumination image enhancement via contrast optimization and color correction. Signal Process. 2018;153:210–20.
13. Ju M, Ding C, Guo YJ, et al. IDGCP: image dehazing based on gamma correction prior. IEEE Trans Image Process. 2019;29:3104–18.
14. Kausar T, Wang M, Idrees M, et al. HWDCNN: multi-class recognition in breast histopathology with Haar wavelet decomposed image based convolution neural network. Biocybern Biomed Eng. 2019;39(4):967–82.
15. Lin C-J, Chu W-L, Wang C-C, et al. Diagnosis of ball-bearing faults using support vector machine based on the artificial fish-swarm algorithm. J Low Freq Noise Vib Active Control. 2020;39(4):954–67.
16. Liu R, Fan X, Zhu M, et al. Real-world underwater enhancement: challenges, benchmarks, and solutions under natural light. IEEE Trans Circuits Syst Video Technol. 2020;30(12):4861–75.

# Chapter 3
# Hair Removal Models

## 3.1 Introduction

The dermatoscopy is a non-invasive diagnostic tool that has gradually expanded its applications from the earliest diagnosis and classification of melanoma to the diagnosis and classification of pigmentary diseases such as nevi, seborrheic keratosis, basal cell carcinoma, vascular tumors, and hemorrhagic lesions. Through reducing the reflection interference of light, dermatoscopy can magnify the local lesions up to 25–150 times or even greater, and observes the skin structure and morphology at the junction of the epidermis, and dermis, and even the superficial layer of the epidermis. Various structures can be seen under the skin microscope, such as pigmented reticular structures, punctate structures, cobblestone structures, "blue-white" veils, degenerative structures, comma shaped blood vessels, and other typical skin disease symptoms.

The early melanoma diagnostic techniques utilize the computer-aided technology to accurately identify specific skin lesions for the clinical evaluation, but there are some drawbacks. For the dermatoscopy images, the low contrast of lesion regions among different skin diseases greatly interferes with the recognition of melanoma, and even the presence of hair in the images further reduces the accuracy of diagnosis. The hair impact on the color, the texture, and boundary features of skin lesions cannot be ignored, and removing hair is an essential precondition on performing skin lesion segmentation and recognition. Removing hair may promote the efficiency of segmentation steps, help experts visually detect the lesion site, and improve diagnostic accuracy.

A group of dermatoscopic images with hair are shown in Fig. 3.1a. The presence of hair can lead to asymmetric and irregular edges, uneven colors, and larger extracted lesion regions. For example, From Fig. 3.1b, it shows that the edges of lesion areas with hair become serrated, and the overall edge shape becomes larger and asymmetrical. At this time, based on the ABCD detection criterion for melanoma [1], some skin diseases, which are originally melanomas, are directly judged as melanoma.



S. Guo et al., *Computer-Aided Intelligent Diagnosis of Skin Melanoma*,
https://doi.org/10.1007/978-981-96-6135-0_3

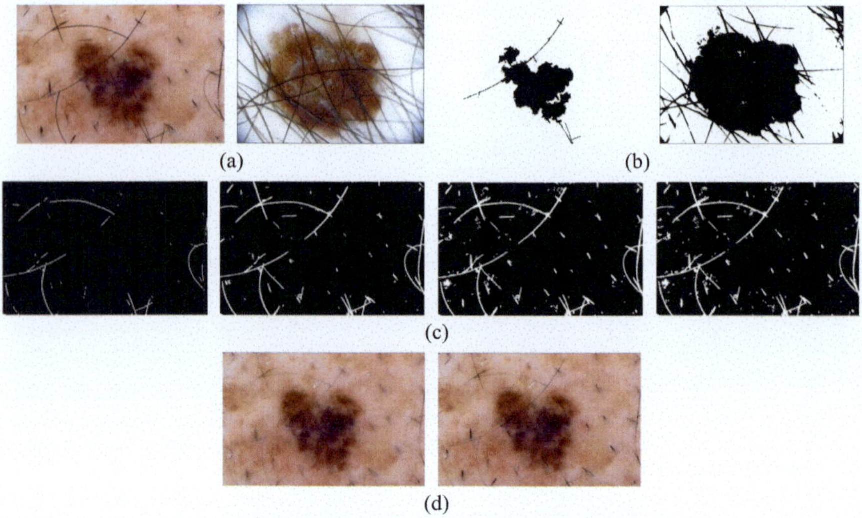


**Fig. 3.1** Hair processing of the dermoscopic images (**a** the original images, **b** the lesion extraction, **c** the threshold adaptation, **d** the residual hair repair)

Therefore, it is necessary to remove hair from dermoscopic images for the accuracy of skin disease detection. It is mentioned that traditional hair extraction and repair algorithms have certain limitations. When extracting hair regions in Fig. 3.1c, it shows that the traditional morphological operations heavily depend on the selected parameters which have a significant impact on the results. It also shows that there unluckily exist the residual hair regions due to the inability to repair the texture of the skin lesion in Fig. 3.1d.

The thresholds [2] or morphological operations [3] directly arise the over-segmentation or the under-segmentation [4]. The over-segmentation can lead to the loss of texture features around the hair, which can result in the loss of important features of some images. The under-segmentation can lead to residual hair information of the image, disrupting the distribution and orientation of features in the overall image. The Criminisi algorithm, as the most classic image texture restoration algorithm, matches sample blocks to the damaged regions in a specific order [5]. Due to the complex computation required in both the priority and the best matching template search during the application process, the computation process takes a considerable amount of time [6]. In response to the above issues, a dermoscopic image hair removal algorithm is proposed based on the maximum inter class variance fuzzy clustering and the improved Criminisi algorithm in this chapter. Firstly, the region growth algorithm to extract discontinuous regions is used; Secondly, the maximum inter class variance fuzzy clustering method is adapted to extract too large regions when the color of hair is close to the surrounding areas; Thirdly, the fuzzy membership function is designed to optimize some difficulties such as easily falling into local optima and poor robustness of hair extraction in clustering; Then, the priority of the traditional Criminisi algorithm is fused with the structural strength and the data coherence features, and simultaneously the color weights are introduced into the sample block matching criteria; Finally, the ant colony algorithm is used to optimize the search path of matching blocks.

## 3.2 The Hair Removal Models

The hair removal models mainly include a hair extraction model based on the maximum inter class variance fuzzy clustering and an image restoration model based on the improved Criminisi. The hair removal models are shown in Fig. 3.2.

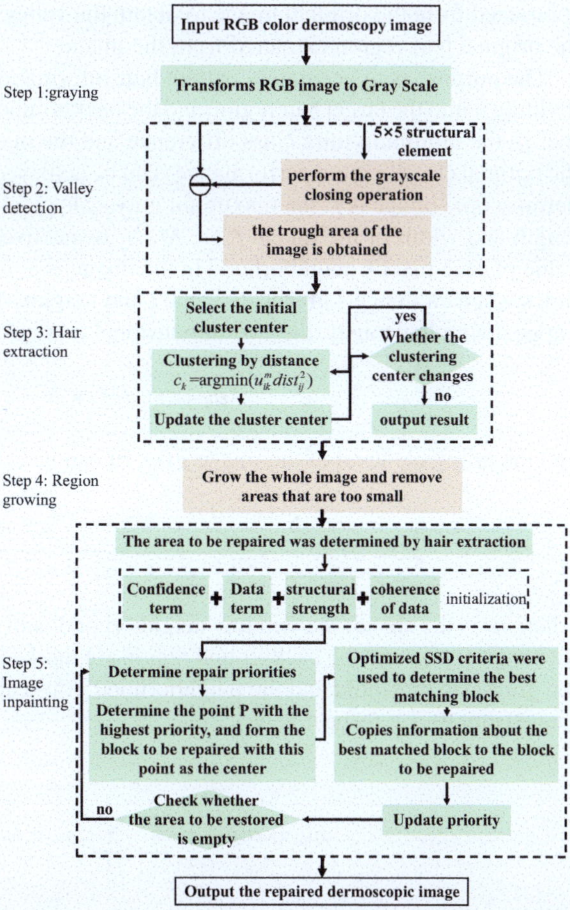


**Fig. 3.2** The flowchart of the hair removal algorithm for dermoscopic images

### 3.2.1 The Hair Extraction Model Based on the Maximum Inter Class Variance Fuzzy Clustering

Due to the fact that the RGB color space contains three channels, it is too complex for directly detecting hair in the RGB color space. Before using the maximum inter class variance fuzzy clustering for hair extraction, the following image preprocessing needs to be completed. The RGB format dermoscopic image is converted into a grayscale image, then valley detection on the dermoscopic image is performed, which is consist of two steps. Firstly, the structural elements are adapted to perform a closure operation on the original image such as expanding, corroding, filling small holes on the object, and connecting adjacent objects, and its main purpose is to preliminarily fill and repair the hair region, and prepare for further hair extraction. Due to the fact that the width of hair in the dermoscopic images is generally less than 10 pixels, the $5 \times 5$ structural elements are adapted to fill the hair region. Then, the closure operation is subtracted from the original image to obtain the valley region of the image, which is the original hair region extracted from the image.

The purpose is to accurately extract hair information from the original image by dividing it into the target hair region and the background region. When these two parts realize the minimum intra class difference and the maximum inter class difference, the optimal classification performances can be achieved. Assuming the preprocessed dermoscopic image is $f$, the maximum grayscale pixel value of the image $f$ is $L$, the length and width of the image $f$ are $M$, $N$, respectively, and the average grayscale value of each pixel's neighborhood in the image is $g$. And $m_{ij}$ denotes the number of times when an image's grayscale value $i$ and neighborhood average grayscale value $j$ appear simultaneously, the two-dimensional joint probability density is defined as

$$p_{ij} = m_{ij}/M \times N \tag{3.1}$$

and the grayscale level of the image $g(m, n)$ can be calculated as

$$g(m, n) = \frac{\sum_{i=-(n_1-1)/2}^{(n_1-1)/2} \sum_{j=-(n_1-1)/2}^{(n_1-1)/2} f(m+i, n+j)}{n_1 \times n_1} \tag{3.2}$$

where $n_1$ is the size of the window neighborhood, and usually takes an odd number; the target region and the background region are marked as $c_b$ and $c_o$; $s$ and $t$ represent the grayscale threshold and the neighborhood grayscale threshold of the image, and range from $[0, L)$, respectively.

Let

$$\omega_b = p(c_b) = \sum_{i=1}^{s} \sum_{j=1}^{t} p_{ij} = \omega_b(s, t) \tag{3.3}$$

$$\omega_o = p(c_o) = \sum_{i=s+1}^{L} \sum_{j=t+1}^{L} p_{ij} = \omega_o(s,t) \tag{3.4}$$

where, $\omega_b$ and $\omega_o$ represent the proportion of non-hair regions and hair regions in the image, respectively. Assuming that the intersected proportion of the different adjacent regions is approximately 0. Therefore, $\omega_b + \omega_o = 1$, which means corresponding vectors of the fur and non-fur regions are

$$\mu_b(s,t) = (\mu_{b1}, \mu_{b2})^T = \left[ \frac{\sum_{i=1}^{s} \sum_{j=1}^{t} i p_{ij}}{\omega_b(s,t)}, \frac{\sum_{i=1}^{s} \sum_{j=1}^{t} j p_{ij}}{\omega_b(s,t)} \right]^T \tag{3.5}$$

$$\mu_o(s,t) = (\mu_{o1}, \mu_{o2})^T = \left[ \frac{\sum_{i=s+1}^{L} \sum_{j=t+1}^{L} i p_{ij}}{\omega_o(s,t)}, \frac{\sum_{i=s+1}^{L} \sum_{j=t+1}^{L} j p_{ij}}{\omega_o(s,t)} \right]^T \tag{3.6}$$

And the overall mean vector is

$$\mu_l(s,t) = (\mu_{l1}, \mu_{l2})^T = \left[ \sum_{i=1}^{L} \sum_{j=1}^{L} i p_{ij}, \sum_{i=1}^{L} \sum_{j=1}^{L} j p_{ij} \right]^T \tag{3.7}$$

The intra class variances of the background and target classes are

$$d_b(s,t) = \sum_{i=1}^{s} \sum_{j=1}^{t} \frac{p_{ij}}{\omega_b(s,t)} (i - \mu_{b1})^2 + \sum_{i=1}^{s} \sum_{j=1}^{t} \frac{p_{ij}}{\omega_b(s,t)} (j - \mu_{b2})^2 \tag{3.8}$$

$$d_o(s,t) = \sum_{i=s+1}^{L} \sum_{j=t+1}^{L} \frac{p_{ij}}{\omega_o(s,t)} (i - \mu_{o1})^2 + \sum_{i=s+1}^{L} \sum_{j=t+1}^{L} \frac{p_{ij}}{\omega_o(s,t)} (j - \mu_{o2})^2 \tag{3.9}$$

and the intra class variance of the intra target class and the background class may be fused as

$$s_w(s,t) = \omega_b(s,t) d_b(s,t) + \omega_o(s,t) d_o(s,t) \tag{3.10}$$

Note: When the fusion of intra class variances is the minimum, the extracted hair region performs the optimal, that is, the optimal segmentation threshold is obtained when Eq. (3.10) reaches to the minimum.

The average inter class variance between the target class and the background class is:

$$s_B(s,t) = \sum_{i=1}^{s}\sum_{j=1}^{t}\omega_b(|i-\mu_{l1}| + |j-\mu_{l2}|) + \sum_{i=s+1}^{L}\sum_{j=t+1}^{L}\omega_o(|i-\mu_{l1}| + |j-\mu_{l2}|) \quad (3.11)$$

Note: When the average inter class variance (3.11) is maximum, the deviation between hair and non-hair regions reaches its maximum, and the hair region extraction effect is the optimal.

Since $s_w(s,t) + s_B(s,t) = s(s,t) = const$, if the intra class variance is the minimum, the inter class variance is the maximum. The objective function is generally solved in enumeration. In order to quickly obtain the minimum threshold vector $(s, t)$ of the designed objective function, it is revealed that solving the objective function can be viewed as a data clustering of a two-dimensional grayscale histogram, where the clustering centers are correspondingly the center of the background region $dot_b$, and the center of the target region $dot_o$. The optimal threshold can be obtained by dividing the given data set into two categories through using fuzzy clustering. The above improved objective function is obtained as follow:

$$J = \min\left[\sum_{k=1}^{L^2}\sum_{i=\{b,o\}} u_{ik}^m dist_{ij}^2\right] \quad (3.12)$$

where, $u_{ik}$ represents the membership function between the data $x_k$ in the two-dimensional grayscale histogram and the $i$th class sample, with a constraint condition $\sum_{i=1}^{2} u_{ik} = 1$; the membership factor $m(m \geq 2)$ generally takes as 2; the $dist_{ik}$ denotes the distance from the data $x_k$ to the cluster center $dot_i$, which is defined as $dist_{ij}^2 = \left(p_{ij}(i,j) - dot_i\right)^2$.

The objective function (3.12) can be solved through using the Lagrangian method, whose solution process is designed as follows:

Step 1: In order to achieve fast classification, the clustering centers of the background and the target regions in the two-dimensional grayscale histogram are selected, for example, the initial clustering centers are selected as $\left(\frac{L}{4}, \frac{L}{4}\right)$ and $\left(\frac{3L}{4}, \frac{3L}{4}\right)$, respectively in the experiment.

Step 2: The distances among each point in the two-dimensional histogram and the two cluster centers are calculated, and the nearest class $c_k$ towards the cluster center $\left(\frac{3L}{4}, \frac{3L}{4}\right)$ is represented as

$$c_k = \operatorname{argmin}\left(u_{ik}^m dist_{ij}^2\right) \quad (3.13)$$

Let the Lagrangian function

$$F = \sum_{i=\{b,o\}} (u_{ik}^m dist_{ik}^2) + \lambda \left( \sum_{i=\{b,o\}} u_{ik} - 1 \right) \tag{3.14}$$

From $\frac{\partial F}{\partial \lambda} = 0$, it gets

$$\frac{\partial F}{\partial \lambda} = \sum_{k=\{b,o\}} u_{ik} - 1 = 0$$

And from $\frac{\partial F}{\partial u_{(i,j)k}} = 0$, it gets

$$\frac{\partial F}{\partial u_{jk}} = m \cdot u_{jk}^{m-1} dist_{ik}^2 - \lambda = 0$$

Further it gets

$$itu_{jk} = \left( \frac{\lambda}{m \cdot dist_{ik}^2} \right)^{\frac{1}{m-1}} = \left( \frac{\lambda}{m} \right)^{\frac{1}{m-1}} \left( \frac{1}{dist_{ik}^2} \right)^{\frac{1}{m-1}} \tag{3.15}$$

Substituting Eq. (3.15) into the constraint conditions to obtain:

$$\sum_{i=\{b,o\}} u_{ik} = \sum_{i=\{b,o\}} \left( \frac{\lambda}{m} \right)^{\frac{1}{m-1}} \left( \frac{1}{dist_{ik}^2} \right)^{\frac{1}{m-1}} = \left( \frac{\lambda}{m} \right)^{\frac{1}{m-1}} \sum_{i=\{b,o\}} \left( \frac{1}{dist_{ik}^2} \right)^{\frac{1}{m-1}} = 1 \tag{3.16}$$

From (3.16), there is

$$\left( \frac{\lambda}{m} \right)^{\frac{1}{m-1}} = \sum_{i=\{b,o\}} \left( \frac{1}{dist_{ik}^2} \right)^{-\frac{1}{m-1}}$$

substituting it into (3.15) to obtain $u_{jk}$

$$u_{ik} = \sum_{i=\{b,o\}} \left( \frac{dist_{jk}}{dist_{ik}} \right)^{-\frac{2}{m-1}}$$

Step 3: The cluster center points of the target and background regions are recalculated as

$$dot_i = \frac{\sum_{x_k \in ck} u_{ik}^m x_k}{\sum_{x_k \in ck} u_{ik}^m} \tag{3.17}$$

Step 4: To determine whether the current cluster centers have moved, if there are any alterations, Steps 2 and 3 are repeated until the given iterated number is reached.

Step 5: The clustering results are output, whose pixels in the two-dimensional grayscale histogram are divided into the following categories, such as the background region denoting the skin lesion and the remaining skin region, and the target region being the hair region.

After the fuzzy clustering segmentation, hair regions have been basically extracted in the image, but due to the fact that only the pixel features of the two-dimensional grayscale histogram are considered in the above processing, its texture features are not taken into account. Therefore, there will be some interferences from dark textures in the extracted skin regions. Further it is needed to remove these relatively coarse and short strips or the dot interferences on the above areas. Here, the region growth algorithm is used to expand and strengthen the extracted hair regions, which can further supplement these regions by combining the texture information around the regions. Then the regional statistics is performed on the extracted connectivity region, and too small regions are removed. For example, the statistical less than 20-pixel regions can always be considered as some interference information in the texture. Back and forth, all hair regions can be extracted.

### 3.2.2 The Improved Criminisi Algorithm for the Hair Repair Model

After extracting the hair regions, it is necessary to repair the obtained region to ensure that the repaired region has similar texture structures with the surrounding skin lesion as much as possible. The Criminisi algorithm is the most commonly used repair algorithm for the image restoration, which repairs the damaged regions by using the intact samples of the image according to the certain priority calculation rules [7].

The repair principles of the improved Criminisi algorithms are presented in Fig. 3.3. Among them, $I$ represents the image regions to be repaired, $\Omega$ does the damaged region, $\Phi$ does the sample region, $\partial\Omega$ represents the intersection between the sample and the damaged region, $\varphi_p$ does the block to be repaired with the centered point $P$ and the size of $9 \times 9$, $n_p$ and $\nabla I_p^{\perp}$ denote the normal direction of $P$ and its isolux line direction, respectively.

When repairing the images, some important steps of the Criminisi algorithm are included as following:

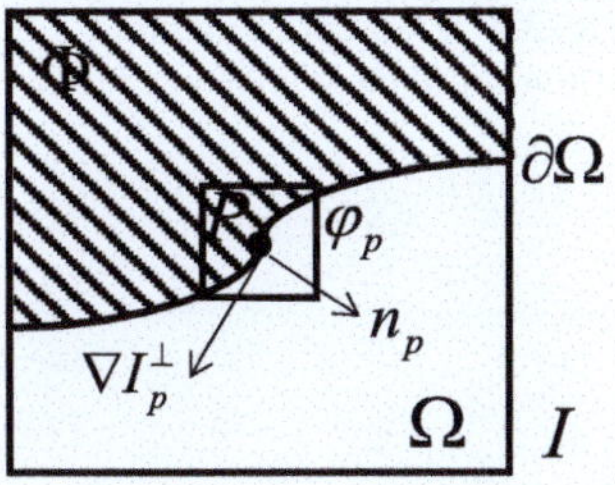


**Fig. 3.3** The repair principle of the improved Criminisi algorithm

(1) The restoration sequence of images is programmed through Eq. (3.18).

$$P(p) = C(p) \times D(p) \tag{3.18}$$

where, $P(p)$ represents the priority of the block to be repaired, $C(p)$ and $D(p)$ denote respectively the confidence term and the data term, and their calculation models are defined as

$$C(p) = \frac{\sum_{q \in \varphi_p \cap \Phi} C(p)}{|\varphi_p|} \tag{3.19}$$

$$D(p) = \frac{\left|\nabla I_p^{\perp} \cdot n_p\right|}{\alpha} \tag{3.20}$$

and $\alpha = 255$ does the normalization parameter.

(2) Based on the sum of squared differences (SSD) criterion, the optimal sample block is obtained through the following calculation method

$$SSD = \arg\min d\left(\varphi_p, \varphi_q\right) \tag{3.21}$$

where $d\left(\varphi_p, \varphi_q\right)$ represents the SSD between the target block and the sample block. According to Eq. (3.21), the sample block, which is the closest to the block to be repaired, is selected in the sample region, and then used to fill the region to be repaired.

(3) The confidence level of the image is updated according to Eq. (3.22):

$$C(p) = C(\hat{p}), \ \forall p \in \varphi_p \cap \Omega \tag{3.22}$$

where $C(p)$ represents the confidence level in the image, $C(\hat{p}) = 0, \ \forall p \in \varphi_p$ and $C(\hat{p}) = 1, \ \forall q \in \varphi_q$ represents the confidence levels for the region to be repaired and the sample region, respectively.

During the image restoration, the regions that need to be repaired are always small and numerous single connected region, and while the traditional Criminisi algorithm is too slow and has the poor repair ability [8–12]. Therefore, the priority level, the

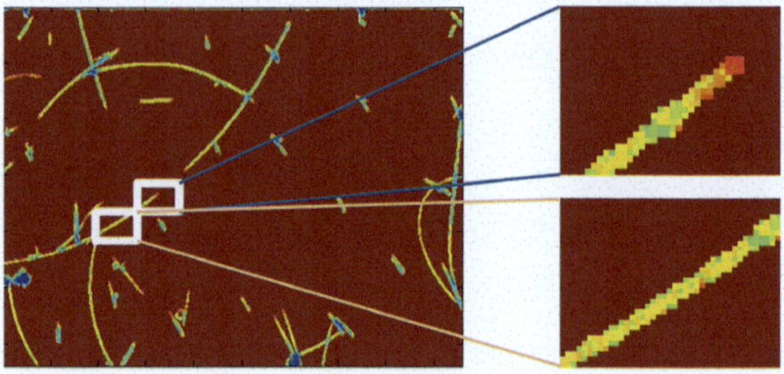

**Fig. 3.4** The representation of the confidence level

repair block distance selections, and the repair paths in the Criminisi algorithm are all improved to complete the algorithm optimization.

For the traditional Criminisi algorithm, the confidence term $C(p)$ and the data term $D(p)$ are directly multiplied to obtain the priority level of the image restoration. The confidence term denotes the number of given pixels in the sample block, which is the proportion of non-hair region; The data term is mainly the inner product of the normal vectors and the isolines, which represents the complexity of linear surface structures. Due to the fact that the regions to be repaired are all needled shapes on the head and relatively flat linear in the middle, there exist at least two types of data terms, as shown in Fig. 3.4. Therefore, the data term cannot uniquely represent the structural features of the regions to be repaired, so the image tensor is introduced. The initial tensor $U^0$ of the image $I$ is defined as:

$$U^0 = \nabla I \cdot \nabla I^T = \begin{bmatrix} I_x^2 & I_x I_y \\ I_x I_y & I_y^2 \end{bmatrix} = \begin{bmatrix} u_{11} & u_{12} \\ u_{21} & u_{22} \end{bmatrix} \tag{3.23}$$

where, $\nabla I = \begin{pmatrix} I_x \\ I_y \end{pmatrix}$ represents the gradient vector of the image $I$, $\cdot$ is the Cartesian inner product, and $I_x$, $I_y$ represents the partial derivatives of the image $I$ along the directions $x$, $y$ respectively. It is clear that $u_{12} = u_{21}$.

For the initial structural tensor $U^0$, the structural tensor $U$ is obtained through the Gaussian convolution after linearly filtering.

$$U = M_p \otimes U^0 = M_p \otimes \begin{bmatrix} I_x^2 & I_{xy} \\ I_{xy} & I_y^2 \end{bmatrix} \tag{3.24}$$

where $M_p$ is a Gaussian kernel and $\otimes$ is a vector accumulation operation.

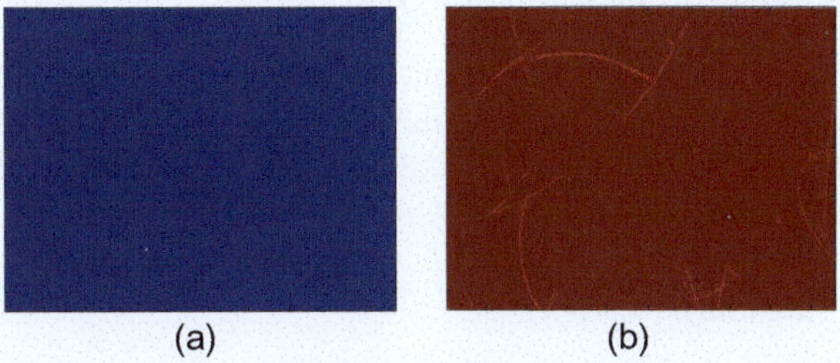

Fig. 3.5 Some features of the structure tensor (**a** the structure strength, **b** the data coherence)

The eigenvalues of a structural tensor $U = \begin{bmatrix} U_{11} & U_{12} \\ U_{21} & U_{22} \end{bmatrix}$ are:

$$\begin{cases} \lambda_1 = \frac{1}{2}\left(U_{11} + U_{22} + \sqrt{(U_{11} - U_{22}) + 4U_{12}^2}\right) \\ \lambda_2 = \frac{1}{2}\left(U_{11} + U_{22} - \sqrt{(U_{11} - U_{22}) + 4U_{12}^2}\right) \end{cases} \tag{3.25}$$

and its structural strength $S_t$ can be calculated by the trace of the structural tensor $U$ as following.

$$S_t = tr(U) = U_{11} + U_{22} = \lambda_1 + \lambda_2 \tag{3.26}$$

and its data coherence is calculated by Eq. (3.27) (Fig. 3.5):

$$H = (\lambda_1 - \lambda_2)^2 \tag{3.27}$$

**Note**: Compared to the data items of the traditional Criminisi algorithm, the structural strength and the data coherence are introduced to describe more image features (to see Fig. 3.5), which can effectively represent the texture shape features of the regions to be repaired.

In order to better integrate different effects on the priority, such as the confidence terms, the data items, the structural strength and the data coherence, the multiplication of priorities is replaced by their addition, whose improved priority calculation equation is defined as:

$$P(p) = C(p) + D(p) + S_t(p) + H(p) \tag{3.28}$$

For example, the SSD criteria of the traditional Criminisi algorithm are as follows:

$$\begin{aligned} &\arg\min d\left(\varphi_p, \varphi_q\right) \\ &= \sum_{I(p)\in\varphi_p, I(q)\in\varphi_q} \left[(I_r(p) - I_r(q))^2 + \left(I_g(p) - I_g(q)\right)^2 + (I_b(p) - I_b(q))^2\right] \end{aligned} \tag{3.29}$$

where there demands the same weight for different color channels. However, in practice, there is a significant deviation in some color channel when passing different color channels. Therefore, the color ratios among different channels needs to be added as different weights to the above SSD criterion, and the improved SSD criterion is revised as

$$\arg\min d(\varphi_p, \varphi_q) = \sum_{I(p)\in\varphi_p, I(q)\in\varphi_q} \left[ (I_r(p) - I_r(q))^2 + c_{rg}\left(I_g(p) - I_g(q)\right)^2 + c_{rb}(I_b(p) - I_b(q))^2 \right] \tag{3.30}$$

where $c_{rb}$ and $c_{rg}$ represent the ratio of the green of be repaired towards the red or the blue of be repaired towards the red, respectively, their specific calculation equation is defined as:

$$C_{kr} = \frac{\sum_{i=1}^{9}\sum_{j=1}^{9}(I_k(i,j) - \mu_k)(I_r(i,j) - \mu_r)}{\sqrt{\sum_{i=1}^{9}\sum_{j=1}^{9}(I_k(i,j) - \mu_k)}\sqrt{\sum_{i=1}^{9}\sum_{j=1}^{9}(I_r(i,j) - \mu_r)}}, k = g, b \tag{3.31}$$

where, $\mu_k(k = g, b)$ represents the mean values of the green (or the blue) and the red channels of the block to be repaired, respectively. By using the above improved matching criterion based on the color ratio, the matching degree among the sample block and the block to be repaired can be more accurately reflected.

The traditional Criminisi algorithm needs a long time to search for the optimal matching block by traversing the entire image. Therefore, the ant colony algorithm is introduced to improve the search path of sample blocks in the Criminisi algorithm [8].

Let $n$, $m$ be the numbers of the sample blocks, the ants, and $d_{ij}(i, j = 1, 2, \ldots, n)$ represents the distance between nodes $i$ and $j$, $\tau_{ij}(t)$ represents the concentration of pheromones between the blocks $i$ and $j$ at $t$ time, and the transfer probability of the ant $i$ selecting the node $j$ is:

$$P_{ij}^{k}(t) = \begin{cases} \frac{\tau_{ij}^{\alpha}(t)[\eta_{ij}(t)]^{\beta}}{\sum_{s\in U_k}[\tau_{is}(t)]^{\alpha}[\eta_{is}(t)]^{\beta}} & j \in U_k \\ 0 & others \end{cases} \tag{3.32}$$

where $U_k$ denotes the next block that ant k is allowed to select; $\alpha$ is the heuristic information factor; $\beta$ is the expected heuristic factor, and generally $\eta_{ij} = 1/d_{ij}$.

When passing one cycle with a certain period $n$, the pheromones of the ant colony on each path are updated as:

$$\tau_{ij}(t + n) = \rho \cdot \Delta\tau_{ij} \tag{3.33}$$

where $\rho$ is the volatilization degree of pheromones; $\Delta\tau_{ij}$ is the increment of pheromones along the path $d_{ij}$ for the entire ant colony, and

$$\Delta\tau_{ij} = \sum_{k=1}^{m} \Delta\tau_{ij}^{k} \tag{3.34}$$

and $\Delta\tau_{ij}^{k}$ denotes the left pheromones on the path $d_{ij}$ for the ant $k$, and

$$\Delta\tau_{ij}^{k} = \begin{cases} Q/L_k & \text{if the } k\text{th ant passing path } d_{ij} \\ 0 & others \end{cases} \tag{3.35}$$

and $Q$ is a constant, $L_k$ represents the distance that the ant $k$ crawls along this path.

The ant colony algorithm in the specific application process are as follows:

Step 1: To initialize $nc$, $\tau_{ij}$ and $\Delta\tau_{ij}^{k}$, an possible ant $k$ $(k = 1, 2, \ldots, m)$ is placed at the starting point of possible $n$ paths;
Step 2: To place the initial starting point of the ant colony $k$ in the current solution set, its probability $P_{ij}^{k}(t)$ is calculated when the ant moves to a node $j$ in the current solution set;
Step 3: The path length $L_k$ $(k = 1, 2, \ldots, m)$ of each ant $k$ is calculated and the corresponding optimal solution in this state is saved;
Step 4: The optimal path is updated, and simultaneously the trajectory intensity is modified;
Step 5: For each side arc $(i, j)$, let $\Delta\tau_{ij} = 0$, $nc = nc + 1$;
Step 6: If the number of iterations $nc$ is less than the predetermined number, then there does not exist the degradation and Step 2 is repeated. Otherwise, the process ends;
Step 7: The current optimal solution is output.

For the block to be repaired, the optimal matching block can be obtained as quickly as possible after the above steps. So, the improved Criminisi hair repair method is shown in Table 3.1.

## 3.3 Experiments and Analysis

### *3.3.1 Dataset and Designed Experiments*

The collected dermatological cases mainly come from the People's Liberation Army General Hospital of China. Due to data limitations, such as insufficient collected cases from the hospital, the rest images are complemented through the ISIC2019 online public dataset. The collected image resolutions range from 637 × 424 to 2556 × 1693, and their contained hair noises are relatively clear, which does not exceed 30% in the dermatoscope image. And more importantly, each image only contains one lesion region. In order to demonstrate the improvement effects of the proposed algorithms in details, three experiment groups are designed in Sects. 3.3.2–3.5.4.

**Table 3.1** The improved Criminisi hair repair method

| Algorithm: The Improved Criminisi hair repair method |
|---|
| **Input**: The dermoscopic image with hair, including the hair region mask;<br>**Output**: The Image after removing hair;<br>1. The image is initialized, and the region of the image to be repaired is determined;<br>2. To repeat Step 2–Step 5<br>3. To calculate the priority of the area to be repaired<br>$P(p) = C(p) + D(p) + S_t(p) + H(p)$;<br>4. To determine the highest priority point P, and to form a block to be repaired around the obtained point;<br>5. To find the optimal sample block based on the SSD criterion combined with the color ratio $\arg\min d(\varphi_p, \varphi_q)$;<br>6. To use the ant colony algorithm to optimize the search paths;<br>7. To replace the region to be repaired with the optimal sample block;<br>8. To update the priority;<br>**9. Until** the remained repair region is empty<br>End; |

**Table 3.2** The characteristics of the used dermatoscopy image data in the experiment

| Image number | Hair proportion (%) | Hair width | Skin lesion | Contrast ratio |
|---|---|---|---|---|
| Image 1 | 1.56 | 6 pixels | Existed | High |
| Image 2 | 3.34 | 17 pixels | Existed | High |
| Image 3 | 3.5 | 9 pixels | Existed | Average |
| Image 4 | 15.02 | 6 pixels | No | Low |
| Image 5 | 4.06 | 7 pixels | No | Low |

For example, the first group evaluates the accuracy of the hair extraction region, the second group does the effects of hair repair, the last group compares the modified Criminisi priority with the traditional ones to demonstrate the improved effects. Five dermoscopic images with typical features for each experiment are selected and their characteristics are presented in Table 3.2.

### 3.3.2 *The Hair Repair Experiment*

Evaluation Indicators

Through comparing with the common hair repair algorithms, including the linear interpolation algorithm [13] (IN), the convolution repair algorithm [14] (CO), and the traditional Criminisi algorithm [7] (TC), the second experiment is mainly to verify the effectiveness of the ant colony optimization Criminisi (AC) algorithm in hair repair. Those parameters in the IN, the CO, and the TC algorithms are retained when their optimal segmentation effects are obtained on multiple experiments. Due to the deletion of standardized hair restoration in dermatoscopy images, many image restoration indicators are no longer practicable. And in order to obtain the standard dermoscopic image restoration, other line segments are manually appended to represent hair on the hairless dermoscopic images. But the above manually appended line segments have significant deficiencies in the pixels and the shape with compared to the realistic scenes. Moreover, when hair regions proportion of the dermatoscopy images is less than 5%, it is more difficult to accurately assess the quality of hair region restoration.

The repair region is generally divided into small 5 * 5 region and compares them with the nearest skin. The evaluation indicators such as the average grayscale value deviation, the grayscale histogram Euclidean distance, the color second-order moment deviation, the Minikovskii distance, and the structural similarity of the two regions are computed or selected. All evaluation indicators except for Minkovski distance are common, the color Minkovski distance is introduced as following. First, the image is converted to the size of 8 * 8 and a 64 level grayscale, and the average grayscale value of all 64 pixels is calculated. Then, the grayscale of each pixel is compared with the obtained average value. For example, the pixel is taken as 1 if the grayscale value is no less than the average value, otherwise the pixel is taken as 0. Finally, a 64-bit integer string is formed.

By contrasting the overall deviation proportion of the formed strings among different images, the Minkovski distance of the images can be introduced as follows.

$$d(x, y) = \sum char_1(i) \oplus char_2(i) \tag{3.41}$$

where $char_1(i)$ and $char_2(i)$ represent the repaired string and the string to be repaired, respectively, and $\oplus$ denotes some exclusive-OR operator.

Experimental Results

For hair repair, some experimental results on five dermatoscopy images are shown in Sect. 3.2. While the comparative results and their evaluation indicators of the extracted regions are correspondingly presented in Figs. 3.6 and 3.7.

For hair repair of all five repaired images, the color features of the regions to be repaired are basically consistent with the surrounding background, but the local details of the image are enlarged. It is well-known that linear interpolation and convolutional methods are based on the pixel values, and it is not possible to realize the texture repair of the hair regions (to see Fig. 3.8b1–b5 and c1–c5), where the texture features of the repaired region are significantly different from the surrounding, and there exists a significant detail loss. Although the traditional Criminisi algorithm can approximately finish the hair repair, but the repaired regions do not match the surrounding colors due to the lack of color features in the designed optimal matching block in Fig. 3.8d1–d5. Through compared among Fig. 3.8d2, e2, and d4 as well as Fig. 3.8e4, it can be found that the improved ant colony optimization Criminisi algorithm has more advantages in hair repairing details. The similarity of the image is directly calculated based on the average grayscale deviation, and a more comprehensive and accurate objective evaluation index is correspondingly realized (to see Fig. 3.9).

It can be clear that the repaired image in Fig. 3.8a5 holds the lowest average pixel deviation by using the improved Criminisi algorithm. The Euclidean distance and the Minkowski distance of the grayscale histogram represent the color features of the image. For example, for the histogram, the smaller is the Euclidean distance, so does the effect, on the contrary, so does the larger Minkovski distance. It can be clear that the color features of the repaired region in Fig. 3.9b and d is effectively upgraded through the improved Criminisi algorithm. The second-order moments and the structural similarity of images represent the texture feature indicators. For example, the smaller is the deviation in the second-order moments, the better does the texture restoration, on the contrary, so does the larger structural similarity. From

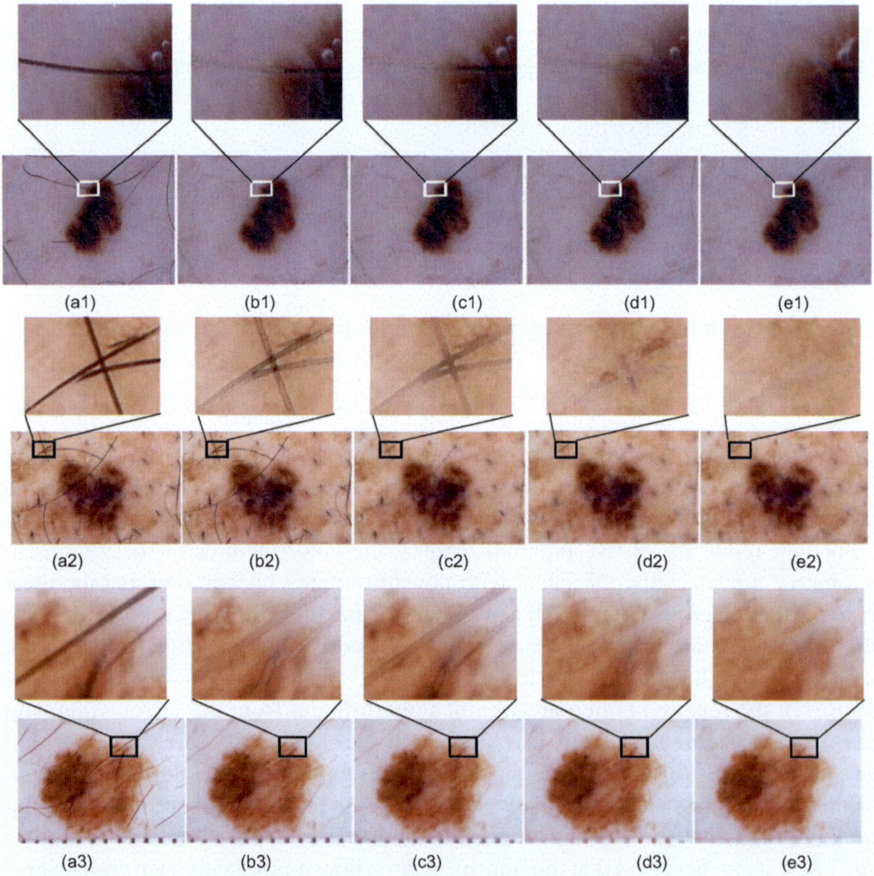


**Fig. 3.6** Dermoscopic image hair restoration experiment results (**a** original image, **b** IN, **c** CO, **d** TC, **e** AC, 1: the 1st image: 2: the 2nd image, 3: the 3rd image, 4: the 4th image, 5: the 5th image)

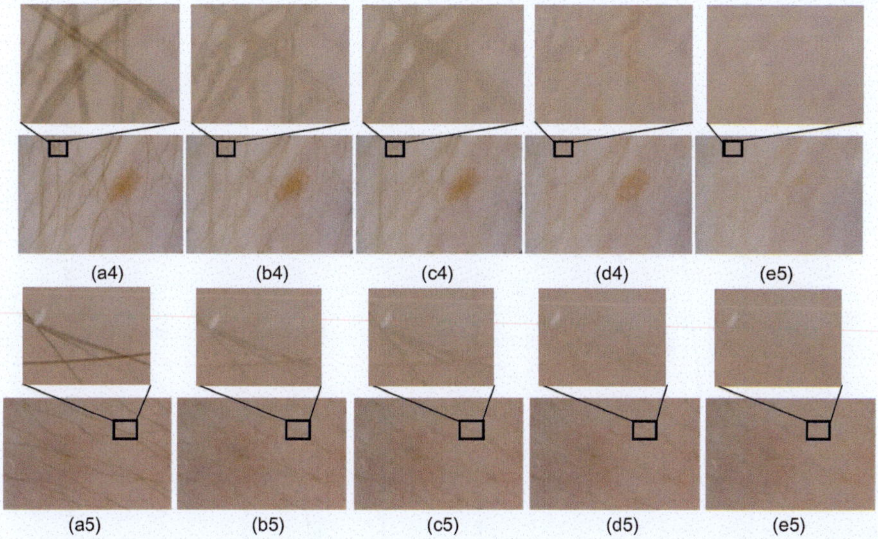


**Fig. 3.6** (continued)

Fig. 3.9c and e, it can be found that compared to the linear interpolation and the convolution algorithms, the improved Criminisi algorithm has better advantages in the image texture restoration.

### *3.3.3 Verification of the Improved Criminisi Algorithm*

The deviations between the original priority and the improved priority for different images are shown in Fig. 3.10. As the continuity of the priority and its rationality cannot be directly observed in two-dimensional images, the three-dimensional images with the priority are further presented in Fig. 3.11. From the above two groups of images, it can be observed that the priority distribution of the repaired region by using the traditional Criminisi algorithm is extremely chaotic and discontinuous, and simultaneously, its corresponding values are small and extremely close. These easily lead to many side effects, for example, it causes the repaired sequences too random, brings some difficulties in continuously repairing a certain region, and even reduces the overall repairing speed. The improved priority enlarges the weight deviation between the priority repairing region and others, brings the weight values of the regions with similar texture structures closer, and makes the distribution of the priority more reasonable, which prove the effectiveness of the improved Criminisi algorithm.

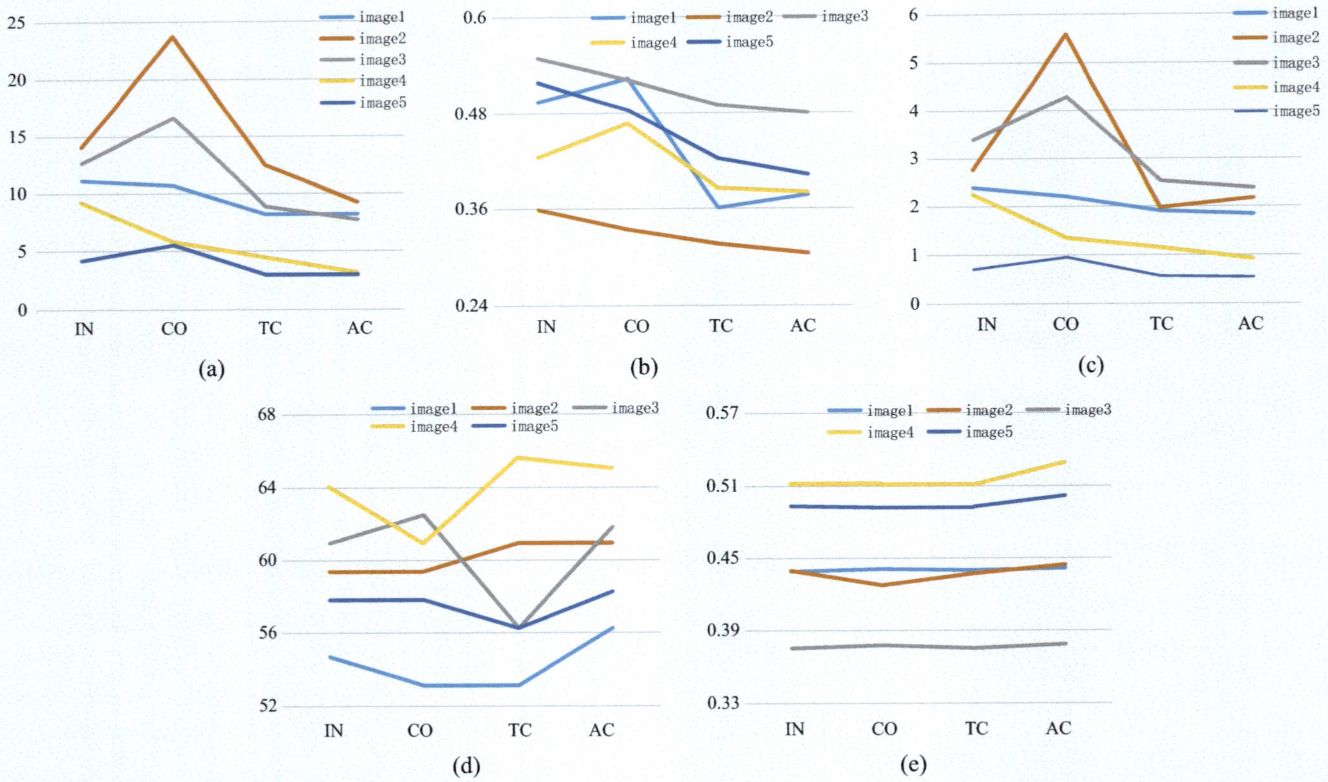


**Fig. 3.7** Evaluation index of experimental results (**a** the average gray value difference, **b** the gray histogram Euclidean distance, **c** the color second moment difference, **d** the Minkovski distance, **e** the structural similarity)

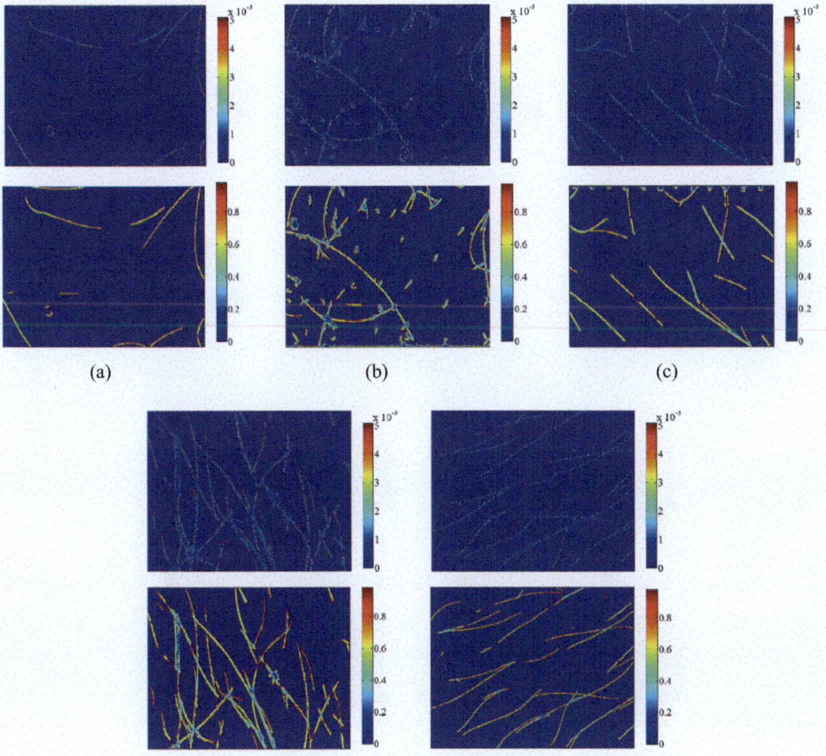

**Fig. 3.8** 2D priority comparison of Criminisi algorithm before and after improvement (**a** the 1st image **b** the 2nd image, **c** the 3rd image, **d** the 4th image, **e** the 5th image)

### 3.3.4 Experimental Analysis

The experimental results of 100 dermoscopic images are presented in this section. Statistical data on the accuracy of extracting hair from 100 images is presented in Table 3.3, while statistical data for all hair repairing experiments is done in Table 3.4. To further demonstrate the practicality of the improved Criminisi algorithm, 24 dermoscopic images with hair are shown in Fig. 3.10, which represent different hair proportions, different hair thicknesses, and different skin colors. After removing hair, the experimental results of dermoscopic images in Table 3.4 are shown through Fig. 3.11. From Tables 3.3 and 3.4, it can be found that the proposed optimized algorithm can increase the accuracy of hair detection about 2–7%, and increase the average accuracy of hair repair about 2–5%. It indicates that these obtained results are well fit with the statistical results of the previous five experiments. More evaluation indicators are analyzed as follows. For example, the proposed hair extraction algorithm can increase the recall, the intersection to union ratio, the accuracy, and the F1 value about 25%, 16%, 24%, and 18% with compared to other algorithms. At

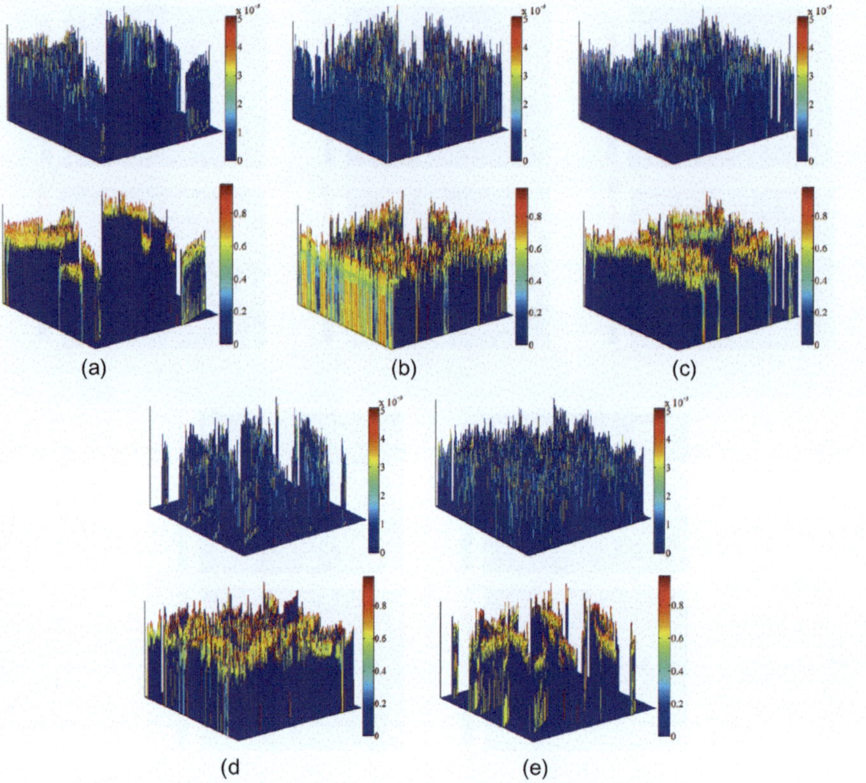


**Fig. 3.9** 3D priority comparison of Criminisi algorithm before and after improvement (**a** the 1st imag**e** **b** the 2nd image, **c** the 3rd image, **d** the 4th image, **e** the 5th image)

the same time, the variance of all data is smaller, which indicates that the proposed optimized algorithm has the optimal stability. The optimized hair repairing algorithm can increase the Minkovski distance about 2% with compared to other algorithms, and can reduce the Euclidean distance, the color second-order moment deviation, and the structural similarity of the grayscale histogram about 38%, 34%, and 28%, respectively. At the same time, the variance of the proposed algorithm is minimized among all algorithms, which indicates its optimal stability. From Fig. 3.11, it can be found that the proposed optimized algorithms perform extremely well in different dermoscopic images, and can repair various dermoscopic images with different hair proportions and different hair thickness.

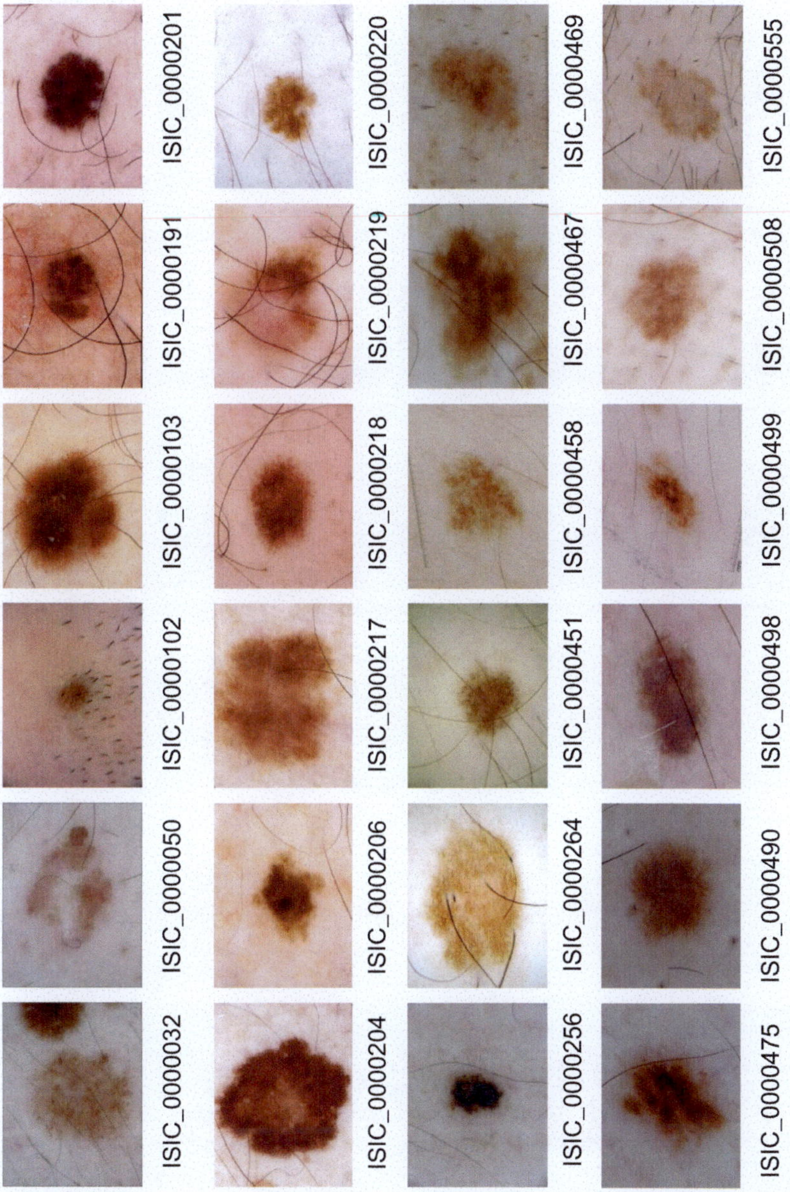


**Fig. 3.10** Typical dermoscopic image with hair

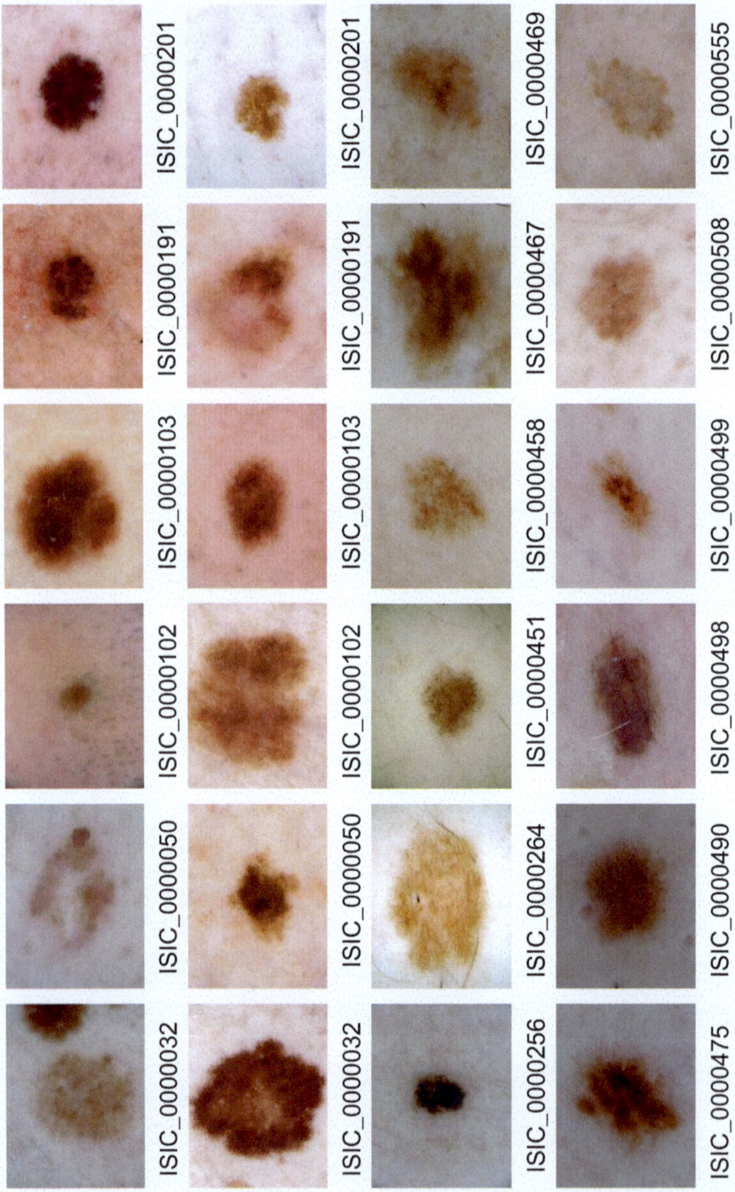


**Fig. 3.11** Results of hair removal experiments from typical dermoscopic images

**Table 3.3** Statistical data of the results of hair extraction experiments

| | PA | | Recall | | MIoU | | Precision | | F1 | |
|---|---|---|---|---|---|---|---|---|---|---|
| | Acc | Var | Acc | Var | Acc | Var | Acc | Var | Acc | Var |
| MO | 0.9607 | 0.0211 | 0.6346 | 0.2140 | 0.6116 | 0.4165 | 0.6133 | 0.3051 | 0.6009 | 0.2641 |
| EO | 0.9680 | 0.0188 | 0.7079 | 0.1622 | 0.5302 | 0.4060 | 0.5254 | 0.2674 | 0.5920 | 0.2468 |
| FC | 0.9160 | 0.0372 | 0.6051 | 0.3990 | 0.5866 | 0.2053 | 0.5626 | 0.2485 | 0.5458 | 0.2004 |
| MT | 0.9668 | 0.0449 | 0.8514 | 0.1209 | 0.6754 | 0.2949 | 0.7017 | 0.1713 | 0.4598 | 0.1834 |
| MFC | 0.9867 | 0.0093 | 0.9500 | 0.0412 | 0.7668 | 0.1177 | 0.8431 | 0.0681 | 0.7333 | 0.0978 |

**Table 3.4** Statistical data of the results of hair repair experiments

| | Difference of average gray value | | Euclidean distance of gray histogram | | Difference of second moment | | Hamming distance | | SSIM | |
|---|---|---|---|---|---|---|---|---|---|---|
| | Acc | Var | Acc | Var | Acc | Var | Acc | Var | Acc | Var |
| IN | 59.3740 | 3.4939 | 10.2667 | 3.8441 | 0.4691 | 0.0769 | 0.4520 | 0.0537 | 2.3059 | 0.9930 |
| CO | 58.7510 | 3.5974 | 12.4827 | 7.7507 | 0.4662 | 0.0779 | 0.4499 | 0.0533 | 2.8807 | 1.9895 |
| TC | 58.4360 | 4.8904 | 7.4061 | 3.7680 | 0.3950 | 0.0658 | 0.4511 | 0.0533 | 1.6295 | 0.7689 |
| AC | 60.4630 | 3.3857 | 6.2443 | 2.9731 | 0.3888 | 0.0629 | 0.4591 | 0.0587 | 1.5751 | 0.8010 |

### *3.3.5 Experimental Discussion*

The hair removal experiments and the validity of the proposed algorithms are carried on through a series of the perfect contrast experiments. The comparative study is crucial for increasing the accuracy of the segmentation or classification for the melanoma and other pigmentary lesions, as is immensely affected by hair cover. Many existed algorithms have not effectively diagnosed the melanoma, and meanwhile, while many existed hair removal algorithms easily interfere with the texture of the lesion, which seriously affects the diagnose quality. The main challenge of hair extraction experiments is how to decrease the interference of the skin lesion region, which easily leads to the extraction region too large or discontinuous. By integrating color and texture features of the image to the greatest extent, some special methods such as the grayscale, the maximum inter class variance fuzzy clustering, and the region growing are designed to remove hair, which improve the accuracy and stability of the hair extraction.

## 3.4 Conclusion

Some challenges, such as discontinuity and insufficient robustness in hair extraction regions, unreasonable priority of traditional hair repair algorithms, insufficient robustness in repair sequences, and color deviation caused by overly simple sample block selection criteria are considered. The hair extraction algorithms based on the maximum inter class variance fuzzy clustering and a Criminisi hair repair algorithm based on ant colony optimization are proposed. Some important contributions are realized, including a qualitative and quantitative proposed evaluation criterion for hair extraction repair algorithms. Based on the proposed criterion, the accuracy of hair detection in the ISIC2019 dataset has increased about 2–7%, and the average accuracy of hair repair about 2–5%. In short, the proposed algorithms have achieved good qualitative and quantitative performances, and obtained a positive balance between the repaired accuracy and the required running time.

## References

1. Congdon NM, Davis CM. A systematic review of the frequency of features of the seven-point checklist in proven cutaneous melanoma: the importance of change. Skin Health Dis. 2023;3(6):295.
2. Nguyen NH, Lee TK, Atkins MS. Segmentation of light and dark hair in dermoscopic images: a hybrid approach using a universal kernel. San Diego: Medical Imaging 2010: Image Processing; 2010. p. 1436–43.
3. Khan AH, Iskandar D, Al-Asad JF, et al. Classification of skin lesion with hair and artifacts removal using black-hat morphology and total variation. Int J Comput Digit Syst. 2021;10:597–604.
4. Loss LA, Bebis G, Parvin B. Iterative tensor voting for perceptual grouping of ill-defined curvilinear structures. Signal Process Lab Swiss Fed Inst Technol Lausanne. 2011;30(8):1503–13.
5. Liu K, Yan H, Meng K, et al. Iterating tensor voting: a perceptual grouping approach for crack detection on el images. IEEE Trans Autom Sci Eng. 2020;18(2):831–9.
6. Ouattara N, Loum GL, Pandry GK, et al. A new image inpainting approach based on Criminisi algorithm. Int J Adv Comput Sci Appl. 2019;10(6):423–33.
7. Yao F. Damaged region filling by improved Criminisi image inpainting algorithm for thangka. Inf Process Visual Technol. 2019;22(6):13683–91.
8. Maheshwari P, Sharma AK, Verma K. Energy efficient cluster based routing protocol for WSN using butterfly optimization algorithm and ant colony optimization. Ad Hoc Netw. 2021;110: 102317.
9. Toossi MTB, Pourreza HR, Zare H, et al. An effective hair removal algorithm for dermoscopy images. Skin Res Technol. 2013;19(3):230–5.
10. Saugeon PS, Guillod J, Thiran JP. Towards a computer-aided diagnosis system for pigmented skin lesions. Signal Process Inst. 2003;27(1):65–78.
11. Schmid P. Segmentation of digitized dermatoscopic images by two-dimensional color clustering. Signal Process Lab Swiss Fed Inst Technol Lausanne. 1999;18(2):164–71.
12. Lee T, Ng V, Gallagher R, et al. Dullrazor®: a software approach to hair removal from images. Cancer Control Res. 1997;27(6):533–43.

13. Kiani K, Sharafat AR. E-shaver: an improved DullRazor® for digitally removing dark and light-colored hairs in dermoscopic images. Cancer Control Res. 2011;41(3):139–45.
14. Li W, Raj ANJ, Tjahjadi T, et al. Digital hair removal by deep learning for skin lesion segmentation. Pattern Recogn. 2021;117:107994.

# Chapter 4
# Interval Segmentation Models

## 4.1 Introduction

Although the maximum inter-class variance fuzzy clustering and the improved Criminisi algorithm can effectively realize the hair removal, but they cannot completely solve the interval extraction caused by the low contrast and the structured noise between hair and skin lesion regions, and there always exists a sticking point of long running time in Fig. 4.1. It is well known that the tensor voting method can extract some salient structural information such as intersections, curves, and surfaces from the image data containing complex interference information through visual perception recognition [1, 2]. Although the tensor voting algorithms can directly obtain the image curve structure in many cases, when the image contrast is too weak or the interference is too strong, it cannot be fully extracted through a single vote and needs to be repeated until the complete curve structure information is obtained [3, 4]. Eggersmann et al. [5] combined tensor voting with iterative voting for the uncertain curve structure of medical cell membranes and obtained good experimental results. For traditional tensor voting algorithms, a fixed size voting domain needs to be determined in advance, which is suitable to specific applications. The size of the voting domain is directly related to the information contents obtained by the voting points. How to select an appropriate voting domain is one of the key issues, so that the voting points can depict the structural distribution of neighboring pixels. When hair regions in images are repaired, the total variation method requires continuous iteration. Designing the appropriate iterations and adjusting the diffusion coefficients to accelerate the iteration running speed is another key issue addressed in the proposed algorithm. Therefore, a dermoscopic image hair removal model is proposed based on the texture spectrum iterative tensor voting and the optimized total variation algorithm. Through considering the texture spectrum of the image, the attenuation function is improved to allow the points on the hair structure to obtain more voting information during the iteration process for more accurate inference of hair structure information. For hair repairing, the prior information of hair noise is firstly modeled

 
S. Guo et al., *Computer-Aided Intelligent Diagnosis of Skin Melanoma*,
https://doi.org/10.1007/978-981-96-6135-0_4

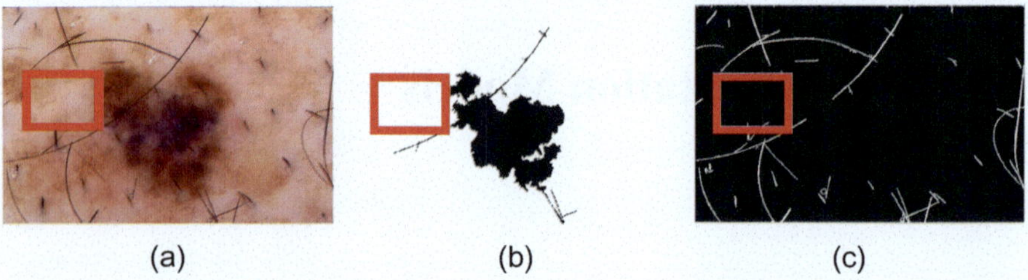


**Fig. 4.1** Hair interval extraction in the dermoscopic images (**a** the original image, **b** the extracted lesion region, **c** the extracted hair structure)

in dermatoscopy images, then an energy functional is established that satisfies the noise constraints, and the diffusion adjustment coefficients are further added into the regularization term, finally the Euler Lagrange model, where the recommended adaptive parameters consistently vary with the iterations, is used to solve the iterative model, and improve the running speed and the quality of image restoration.

## 4.2 Hair Removal Model

Based on the texture spectrum iterative tensor voting and the optimized total variation, the proposed hair removal model includes a hair extraction model and a total variation image restoration model, to see Fig. 4.2.

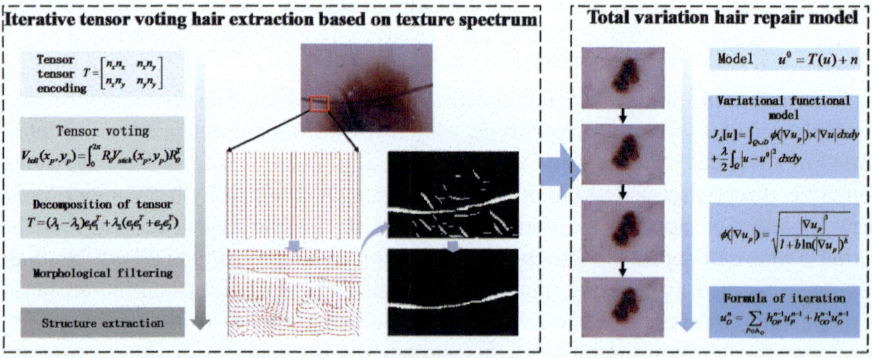


**Fig. 4.2** The proposed hair removal model

### 4.2.1 Hair Extraction Model Based on the Texture Spectrum Iterative Tensor Voting

The tensor voting algorithm generally extracts some salient structural information from the images with complex interference, including the following four steps such as tensor encoding, tensor voting, tensor decomposition, and structural extraction [5].

Tensor encoding is the process of arranging the position and direction of input information into a tensor form. When the input structure has no direction, it can be encoded into a spherical tensor form of feature values $\lambda_1 = \lambda_2 = 1$ as follows

$$T = \begin{bmatrix} 1 & 0 \\ 0 & 1 \end{bmatrix} \tag{4.1}$$

When the input information contains the direction $\vec{n}(n_p, n_p)$, it can be described with a following bar tensor form of eigenvalues $\lambda_1 = 1, \lambda_2 = 0$.

$$T = \begin{bmatrix} n_x n_x & n_x n_y \\ n_x n_y & n_y n_y \end{bmatrix} \tag{4.2}$$

After encoding, each tensor transmits its own information to the other tensors in the voting domain, and further infers the overall structure by accepting the voting information of the other tensors.

Taking Fig. 4.3a for an example, there exists a bar tensor $T = e_0 e_0^T$ at $(x_0, y_0)$, where $e_0 = \begin{bmatrix} 0 & 1 \end{bmatrix}^T$, and the voting information $V_{stick}(x_p, y_p) = F \times e_p e_p^T$ is generated by the bar tensor at a point $(x_p, y_p)$ where $F$ is the decay function, and $e_p$ is the unit vector.

The direction estimation of $e_p$ and the attenuation function $F$ are defined as

$$\begin{cases} e_p = e_0[-\sin(2\theta), \cos(2\theta)]^T \\ F(s, k, \sigma) = e^{-\left(\frac{s^2 + ck^2}{\sigma^2}\right)} \end{cases} \tag{4.3}$$

where, $s$ and $L$ represent the length and the distance between $(x_p, y_p)$ and $(x_0, y_0)$, respectively, $s = \theta L / \sin(\theta)$, $k = 2\sin(\theta)/L$ are curvatures of the close arc, a control parameter C is used to balance the distance and the curvature, the scaling factor $\sigma$ is controlled through the rate of voting decay, and $l$ is related to the size of the voting domain as following

$$e^{-\frac{l^2}{\sigma^2}} = 0.01 \tag{4.4}$$

and the corresponding voting field of the stick tensor is shown in Fig. 4.3b.

More importantly, the voting information of the spherical tensor at $(x_p, y_p)$ can be obtained as

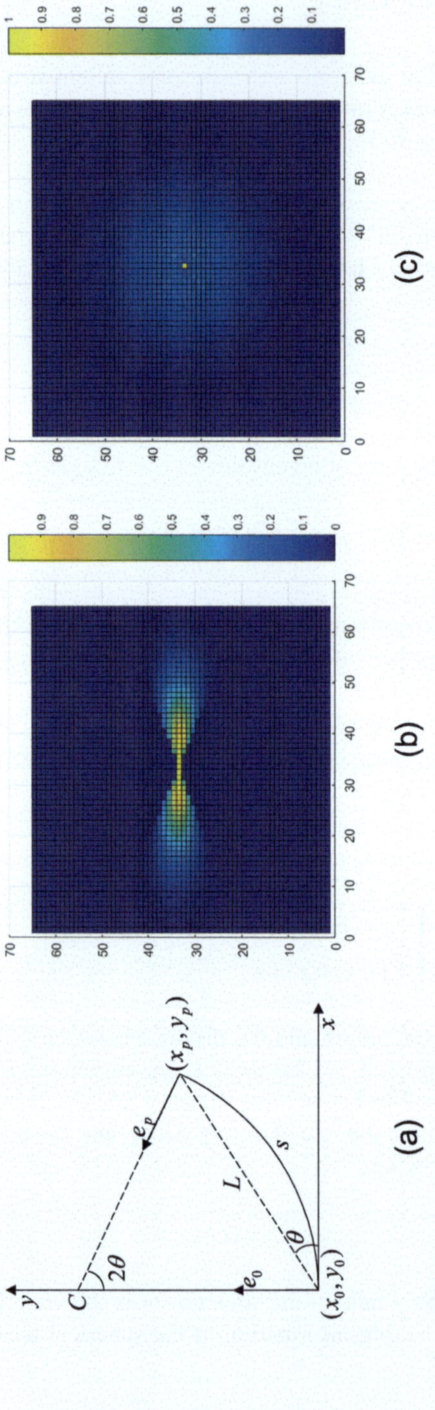


**Fig. 4.3** Schematic diagram of tensor voting field (**a** point-to-point voting, **b** rod tensor voting, **c** ball tensor voting)

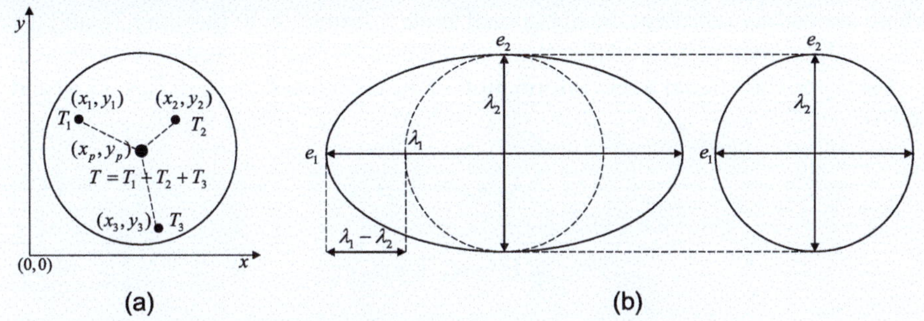


**Fig. 4.4** Schematic of tensor voting (**a** tensor voting, **b** tensor decomposition)

$$V_{ball}(x_p, y_p) = \int_0^{2\pi} R_\theta V_{stick}(x_p, y_p) R_\theta^T \tag{4.5}$$

where $R_\theta$ represents the angle transformation matrix. The voting ground is shown in Fig. 4.3c.

During the voting process, the point $(x_p, y_p)$ will linearly accumulate the votes casted by the point $(x_i, y_i)$ to generate a new tensor within the voting domain, as shown in Fig. 4.4a. The spherical tensor and the rod tensor can be obtained through decomposing the above tensor, and further its directional structural characteristics are inferred in Eq. (4.6).

$$T = (\lambda_1 - \lambda_2)e_1 e_1^T + \lambda_2(e_1 e_1^T + e_2 e_2^T) \tag{4.6}$$

In Fig. 4.4b, the feature diagrams are obtained after tensor decomposition, whose directions are described as $(e_1 e_1^T + e_2 e_2^T)$ and $e_1 e_1^T$, respectively.

It is well-known that the information of the tensor itself will change after a vote, but a single vote cannot fully infer the structural information of the point. It is necessary to continuously improve the voting results through some iterative methods.

Through integrating the texture spectrums, an efficiently iterative tensor voting algorithm is proposed as follows.

First, the grayscale value $I_{xy}$ in the input point $(x, y)$ is encoded as

$$T_{xy} = \begin{bmatrix} (255 - I_{xy})/255 & 0 \\ 0 & (255 - I_{xy})/255 \end{bmatrix} \tag{4.7}$$

Then, the iterative voting will be conducted on the image. The directional angle difference $\beta$ between the voter and receiver is calculated using Eq. (4.8).

$$\beta = |\alpha_A - \alpha_B| \tag{4.8}$$

where, $\alpha_A$ and $\alpha_B$ represent the directional angle information of the voter $T_A$ and the receiver $T_B$, respectively. And the improved attenuation function further is calculated.

Third, the directional angle information of $T_A$ is obtained through Eqs. (4.9) and (4.10)

$$T_A = \lambda_{a1}e_{a1} + \lambda_{a2}e_{a2} \tag{4.9}$$

$$e_{a2} = (\cos\alpha_A, \sin\alpha_A) \tag{4.10}$$

and the directional angle information of $T_B$ is obtained through Eqs. (4.11) and (4.12)

$$T_B = \lambda_{b1}e_{b1} + \lambda_{b2}e_{b2} \tag{4.11}$$

$$e_{b2} = (\cos\alpha_B, \sin\alpha_B) \tag{4.12}$$

For the traditional algorithms, the size of the voting domain is generally fixed, but a large modelling analysis shows that the size of the voting field should proportionally decrease according to the correlation among each pixel and its surrounding pixels. Therefore, the texture spectrum is adapted to represent this correlation. The 5 × 5 neighborhood is defined as a texture primitive for the pixel $P$, and $Vp_i(i = 1, 2, \ldots, 25)$ is used to represent the deviation between the texture primitive and the center pixel, and

$$Vp_i = \begin{cases} 0, \ if \ \left|I_i - I_p\right| \le T_1 \\ 1, \ if \ T_1 \le \left|I_i - I_p\right| \le T_2 \\ 2, \ \text{others} \end{cases} \tag{4.13}$$

where $T_1$ and $T_2$ are the threshold constants of the image, $T_2 = G/2$, $T_1 = 2$ are taken in the experiment, and $G$ is the grayscale level.

For the pixel points $P$, the texture spectrum parameter $Vp$ is defined as

$$Vp = \frac{1}{25}\sum_{i=1}^{25} Vp_i \tag{4.14}$$

And then the impact of image texture on the scale parameters of the voting field is described as $\sigma = f(Tx(M))$.

For example,

$$Tx(M) = \frac{1}{m \times n}\sum_{i=1}^{n}\sum_{j=1}^{m} V_{ij} \tag{4.15}$$

and $V_{ij}$ is the texture spectrum of the point $(i, j), f(\cdot)$ is taken as the inverse scaling function, and $k$ is chose as the adjustment coefficient, then

$$\sigma = k \cdot \frac{1}{Tx(M)} = \frac{kmn}{\sum_{i=1}^{n}\sum_{j=1}^{m} V_{ij}} \tag{4.16}$$

And then, the new attenuation function in this chapter is adapted as Eq. (4.17):

$$DF(s, k, \sigma) = e^{-\left(\frac{s^2 + ck^2 + c_1\beta}{\sigma^2}\right)} \tag{4.17}$$

where $c_1$ denotes a fixed constant used to adjust the attenuation function.

Once the directional angle of the voter changes very little, the above iteration process stops. The voter directional angle during the two iterations is calculated through Eq. (4.18):

$$\theta^i = \sum_{n=1}^{N} \left|\alpha_n^i - \alpha_n^{i-1}\right| / n \tag{4.18}$$

where, $N$ represents the number of voting points and $\alpha_n^i$ represents the direction information of the $i$th tensor during the next vote. Once $\theta^i$ is less than the given threshold, the above iterations finish.

The above texture spectrum iterative tensor voting algorithm is used to extract hair information, whose overall process is shown in Table 4.1. Many simulation details on initialization encoding and iterative voting are presented in Fig. 4.5. An example of the changes in tensor during the voting process is shown in Fig. 4.6, where the proposed algorithm's ability in handling structured noise is demonstrated in 4.6a and b. Due to the similar texture structure of the lesion area with the hair, the initial extracted region contains a large amount of pseudo information. As further iterating, the lesion region on the background is gradually eliminated, and the structure information of the hair becomes clearer. From 4.6a and c, it demonstrates the algorithm's iteration ability in extracting the hair intervals, which are repaired as the algorithm continuously runs. As the extracted image still has the influence of skin lesion area, some morphological filtering methods are added to remove the residual noise, and it is shown in Fig. 4.7 that the interference is filtered out while the hair structure is well preserved.

### 4.2.2 *Total Variational Image Restoration Models with Optimizing Diffusion Adjustment Coefficients*

The variational techniques for image restoration requires the degradation image modelling [6]. Assuming that the hair is artificially added as noise information,

**Table 4.1** The iterative voting method based on texture spectral tensors

| Algorithm: The iterative voting method based on texture spectrum tensor |
|---|
| **Input**: the dermoscopic images with hair information;<br>**Ouput:** the hair structure of the image;<br>1. To grayscale the image and perform the inversion operation;<br>2. To perform initialization encoding on pixels;<br>**3. Repeat**<br>4. Tensor votes $V_{ball}(x_p, y_p) = \int_0^{2\pi} R_\theta V_{stick}(x_p, y_p) R_\theta^T d\theta$;<br>5. To calculate the deviation of iteration angles $\theta^i = \sum_{n=1}^{n=N} \lvert\alpha_n^i - \alpha_n^{i-1}\rvert / n$;<br>**6. Until** $\theta^i$ < threshold **or** the maximum number of iterations reaches<br>7. Tensor decomposes $T = (\lambda_1 - \lambda_2)e_1e_1^T + \lambda_2(e_1e_1^T + e_2e_2^T)$;<br>8. To perform the morphological filtering operation;<br>End; |

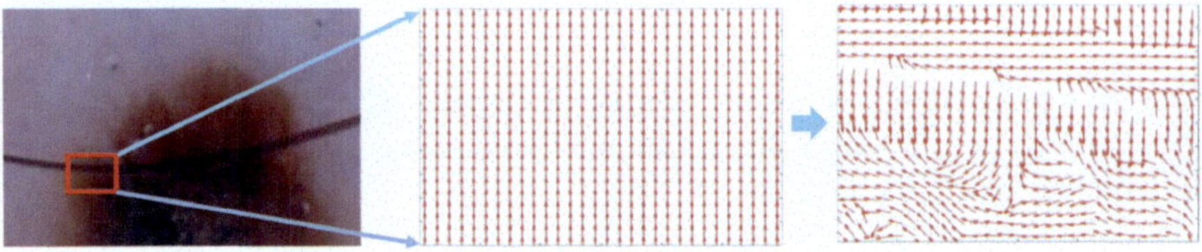

(a) (b) (c)

**Fig. 4.5** Initial tensor and spherical voting results (**a** original image, **b** distribution of eigenvectors of initial tensor, **c** distribution of eigenvectors of tensor after spherical voting)

the degradation model of the dermoscopic image is shown as

$$u^0 = T(u) + n \tag{4.19}$$

where, $u$ denotes the initial value of the image without fur noise, $u^0$ does the observed image, the additive noise $n$ refers to the hair information of the image, and the degradation function $T$ represents a series of operations during the image acquisition process, which often reduce the clarity of the image. For the imaging process, the goal of image restoration can be considered as modelling the prior information to infer a pure image.

Based on the total variational methods for image restoration, an energy functional, which satisfies noise constraints, is firstly established.

$$J_\lambda[u] = \int_{Q \cup D} \phi(\lvert\nabla u_p\rvert) \times \lvert\nabla u\rvert dxdy + \frac{\lambda}{2} \int_Q \lvert u - u^0\rvert^2 dxdy \tag{4.20}$$

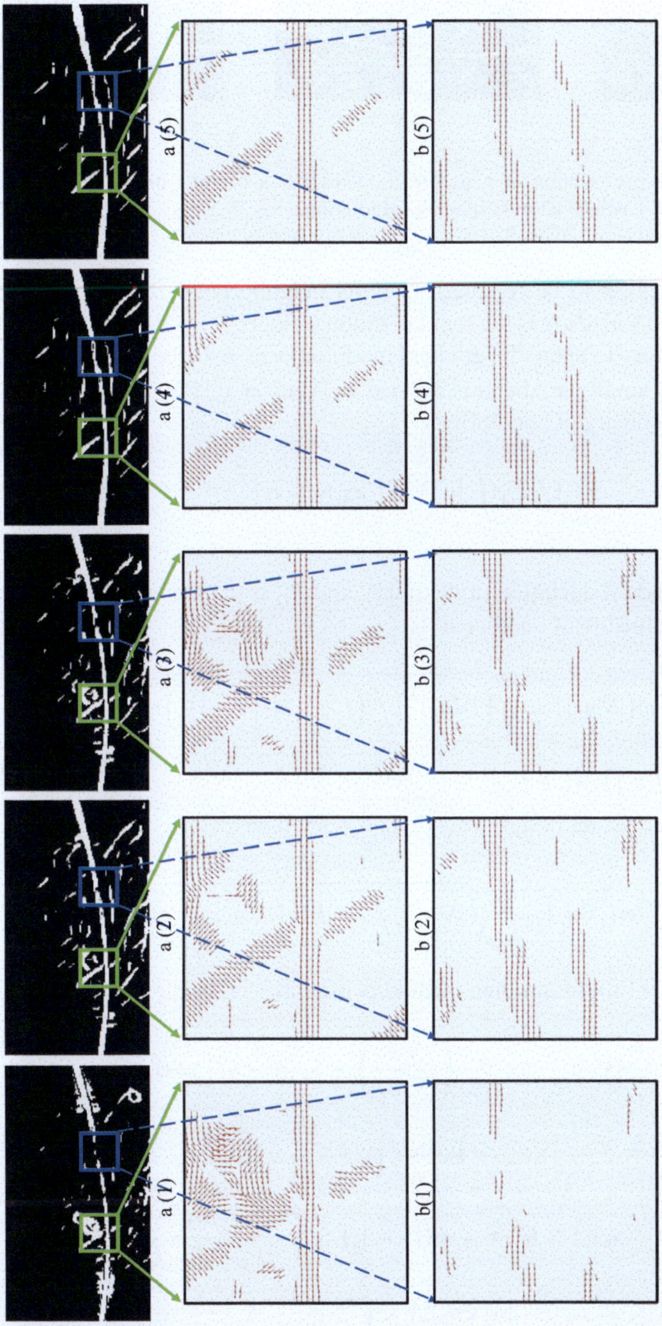


**Fig. 4.6** Schematic diagram of the iterative process of hair extraction (**a** binarization results of the rod saliency map during iteration, **b** feature vector distribution in the green box, **c** feature vector distribution in the blue box)

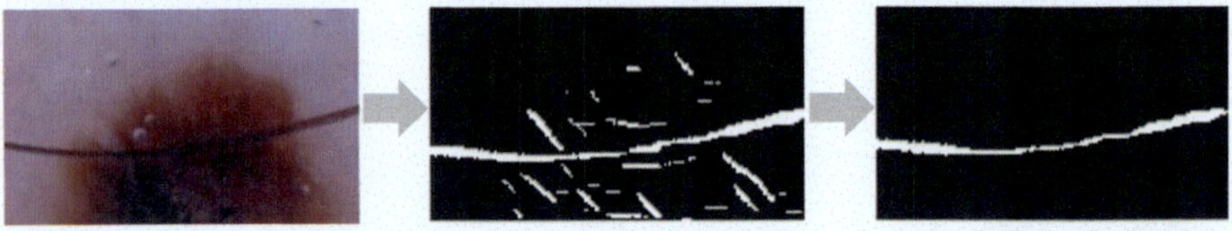


**Fig. 4.7** Schematic representation of hair extraction results (**a** original image, **b** results after iterative tensor voting, **c** results after morphological filtering)

where, $D$ is the region to be repaired, $Q$ is its neighborhood, $\lambda$ is the Lagrange multiplier, $\int_{Q\cup D}\phi(|\nabla u|)dxdy$ is the regularization term, $r(|\nabla u|) = |\nabla u|$, and $|\nabla u|$ is the gradient modulus. To avoid the gradient modulus $|\nabla u| = 0$, the gradient modulus with adding a very small parameter is defined as $|\nabla u|_\varepsilon = \sqrt{|\nabla u|^2 + \varepsilon^2}$.

The hair noise constraint condition is

$$1/A_Q \int\limits_Q |u - u^0|^2 dxdy = \sigma^2$$

where $\sigma$ is the standard deviation of the noise, and $A_Q$ is the area of $Q$.

The diffusion adjustment coefficient is

$$\phi(|\nabla u_p|) = \sqrt{\left(|\nabla u_p|^3\right) / \left(l + b\ln(|\nabla u_p|)^k\right)} \tag{4.21}$$

where $b \in (0, 1)$, $l \in [1, 4]$, $k > 1$.

To avoid $|\nabla u_p| = 0$, let $|\nabla u_p|_\delta = \sqrt{|\nabla u_p|^2 + \delta^2}$, then

$$\phi(|\nabla u_p|_\delta) = \sqrt{|\nabla u_p|_\delta^3 / l + b\ln(|\nabla u_p|_\delta)^k} \tag{4.22}$$

For obtaining $u$, the Euler Lagrange method is used as

$$-\phi(|\nabla u_p|_\delta) \times \nabla \cdot \left(\frac{\nabla u}{|\nabla u|_\delta}\right) + \lambda_z(u - u^0) = 0 \tag{4.23}$$

Let $v = (v^1, v^2) = \nabla u / |\nabla u|_\delta$, it further gets

$$\begin{aligned}\phi(|\nabla u_p|_\delta) \times \nabla \cdot v &= \phi(|\nabla u_p|_\delta) \times \left(\frac{\partial v^1}{\partial x} + \frac{\partial v^2}{\partial y}\right) \\ &\approx \phi(|\nabla u_p|_\delta) \times \left(\frac{v_e^1 - v_w^1}{h} + \frac{v_n^2 - v_s^2}{h}\right)\end{aligned} \tag{4.24}$$

where $h$ is the step size.

Taking $h = 1$ and the point $e$ as an example, then

$$\begin{aligned}\phi(|\nabla u_e|_\delta) \times v_e^1 &\approx \sqrt{\frac{|\nabla u_e|_\delta^3}{l + b\ln(|\nabla u_e|_\delta)^k}} \times \frac{1}{|\nabla u_e|_\delta}\left(\frac{u_E - u_O}{h}\right) \\ &= \sqrt{\frac{|\nabla u_e|_\delta}{l + b\ln(|\nabla u_e|_\delta)^k}} \times \left(\frac{u_E - u_O}{h}\right)\end{aligned} \tag{4.25}$$

further,

$$0 = \sum_{P\in\Lambda_O} \sqrt{\frac{|\nabla u_p|_\delta}{l + b\ln\left(|\nabla u_p|_\delta\right)^k}} \times (u_O - u_P) + \lambda_z\left(u_O - u_O^0\right) \tag{4.26}$$

then

$$w_P = \sqrt{\frac{|\nabla u_p|_\delta}{l + b\ln\left(|\nabla u_p|_\delta + \delta\right)^k}} \tag{4.27}$$

where the added parameter δ is to avoid $|\nabla u_p|_\delta = 0$.

Further, the weight coefficients are designed as

$$h_{OP} = \frac{w_P}{\sum_{P\in\Lambda_O} w_P + \lambda_z}, \quad h_{OO} = \frac{\lambda_z}{\sum_{P\in\Lambda_O} w_P + \lambda_z} \tag{4.28}$$

then

$$u_O = \sum_{P\in\Lambda_O} h_{OP} u_P + h_{OO} u_O^0 \tag{4.29}$$

Last, the obtained iterative equation is

$$u_O^n = \sum_{P\in\Lambda_O} h_{OP}^{n-1} u_P^{n-1} + h_{OO}^{n-1} u_O^{n-1} \tag{4.30}$$

**Note:** For the initial iteration stage of Eq. (4.30), a smaller value $\delta$ is taken to ensure larger diffusion coefficients and an accelerated diffusion speed, while for the end of the iteration, the edge information is maintained through increasing $\delta$ and reducing the diffusion coefficients to improve the visual effect of the repaired image.

The hair repair through the total variation method with optimized diffusion adjustment coefficients is shown in Table 4.2.

**Table 4.2** The total variational image restoration for optimizing diffusion adjustment coefficients

| Algorithm: The Total Variational Image Restoration with Optimized Diffusion Adjustment Coefficients |
|---|
| **Input**: The dermoscopic images with hair, and the hair region masks;<br>**Ouput**: the dermoscopic images after removing hair;<br>1. To establish an image degradation model $u^0 = T(u) + n$;<br>2. a functional model is constructed, which satisfies noise constraints<br>$J_\lambda[u] = \int_{Q \cup D} \phi(\|\nabla u_p\|) \times \|\nabla u\| dxdy + \frac{\lambda}{2} \int_Q \|u - u^0\|^2 dxdy;$<br>**3. Repeat**<br>4. To solve the model $u_O^n = \sum_{P \in \Lambda_O} h_{OP}^{n-1} u_P^{n-1} + h_{OO}^{n-1} u_O^{n-1}$;<br>**5. Until** the maximum number of iterations is reached<br>End |

## 4.3 Experiments and Analysis

The dataset and experimental environments in this chapter are consistent with those in Chap. 3. Some important experiments such as the hair extraction evaluation, the optimization validation of the proposed total variation method, the hair repair evaluation, and the evaluation of its melanoma recognition rate are designed. For the first three groups of experiments, detailed comparative experiments are designed using five images with hair under complex background interferences, some of whose features are presented in Table 4.3, and for the fourth experiment, more additional data are used to validate the recognition of melanoma.

### *4.3.1 Hair Extraction Evaluation Experiment*

The proposed texture spectrum iterative tensor voting algorithm in hair extraction is validated, and simultaneously the comparison of its performances with some existed algorithms in this field is also presented. Those existed algorithms [7–9] include the morphological operation + threshold segmentation (MT), the edge operator (EO), the

**Table 4.3** Dermatoscopy image data information

| Image Number | Hair proportion (%) | The proportion of hair in the affected region (%) | Hair width ( pixels) |
|---|---|---|---|
| Image 1 | 1.89 | 21 | 6 |
| Image 2 | 3.34 | 19.9 | 17 |
| Image 3 | 2.96 | 36.7 | 6 |
| Image 4 | 2.01 | 39 | 7 |
| Image 5 | 1.46 | 33.9 | 5 |

fuzzy clustering (FC), the maximum variance fuzzy clustering (MFC) method. The results of five sets of hair extraction experiments are directly displayed in Fig. 4.8, and their objective evaluation indicators are also provided for the experimental results in Fig. 4.9. In particular, the objective evaluation indicators, the experimental data settings, and the parameter selection methods used in the experiment are the same as those in Sect. 3.3.2.

It can be intuitively shown that compared to the other comparison algorithms in the experiments, the texture spectrum iterative tensor voting algorithm effectively solves the following extraction interval problems, such as the low contrast between hair and skin lesion regions, the pseudo hair phenomenon caused by complex backgrounds. The hair extraction performances, which are comparative with the four algorithms in five groups of dermoscopic images, are shown in Fig. 4.8b–e, and it can be easily shown that other four algorithms have obvious shortcomings during extracting hair. It is well-known that extracting hair depends so heavily on the selected thresholds, and too large or too small thresholds easily result in low accuracy of the extracted region. So, morphological operations need to combine with threshold segmentation, and preliminarily extract hair according to the size of pixels. Due to the certain width limit of hair regions, the edge operators can only extract their edges and are difficulty in directly separating hair regions; The fuzzy clustering method directly divides the image into different regions, one of which is the extracted hair region. This method is relatively convenient, but it takes a long time and there exist some difficulties in distinguishing hair regions from skin lesion regions with similar pixel values; Although the maximum inter class variance fuzzy clustering can effectively solve the above difficulties, it still cannot effectively solve the extraction interval problem caused by low contrast between hair and skin lesion regions. From Fig. 4.8f1–f5, it can be shown that the proposed texture spectrum iterative tensor voting algorithm efficiently overcomes the above difficulties in fully extracting hair intervals of the dermoscopic images. It can be seen from the qualitative evaluation indicators in Fig. 4.9 that the proposed method preferably performs in the pixel accuracy, the recall, the intersection to union ratio, and F1 value among all types of images. It should be emphasized that the average classification accuracy of hair and skin lesion regions already reaches to 99.28%, and the accuracy of hair recognition exceeds 95%, which are all far beyond the corresponding recognition rates of other four algorithms.

### 4.3.2 Optimization Experiment of Total Variation Method

In order to improve the repair speed and the repair quality of dermoscopic images, diffusion adjustment coefficients are introduced to the regularization term, and adaptive parameters that vary with the iterations are designed to dynamically adjust the diffusion speed of the iteration process. When repairing Image 1, the convergences of the means of the four diffusion coefficients of the original and improved algorithms are intuitively demonstrated in Fig. 4.10, where $w_{E1}, w_{N1}, w_{W1}, w_{S1}$ denote

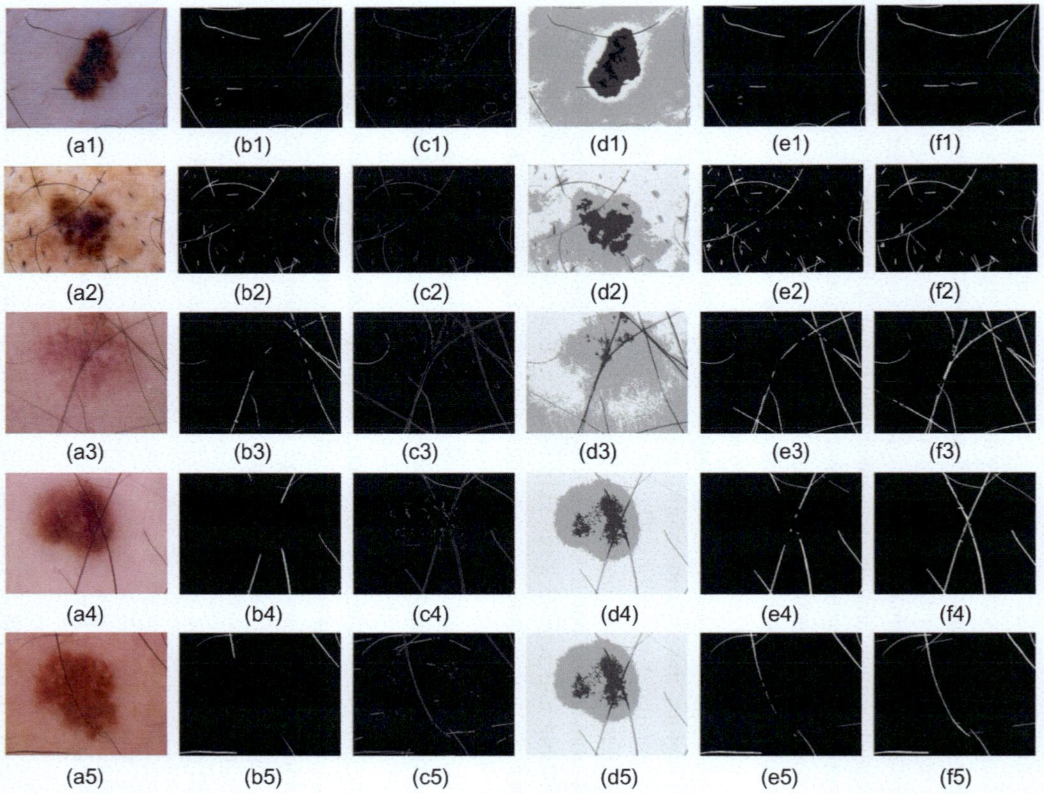


**Fig. 4.8** Results of hair extraction experiment (**a** original image, **b** MT, **c** EO, **d** FC, **e** MFC, **f** TS-ITV, 1: image 1, 2: image 2, 3: image 3, 4: image 4, 5: image 5)

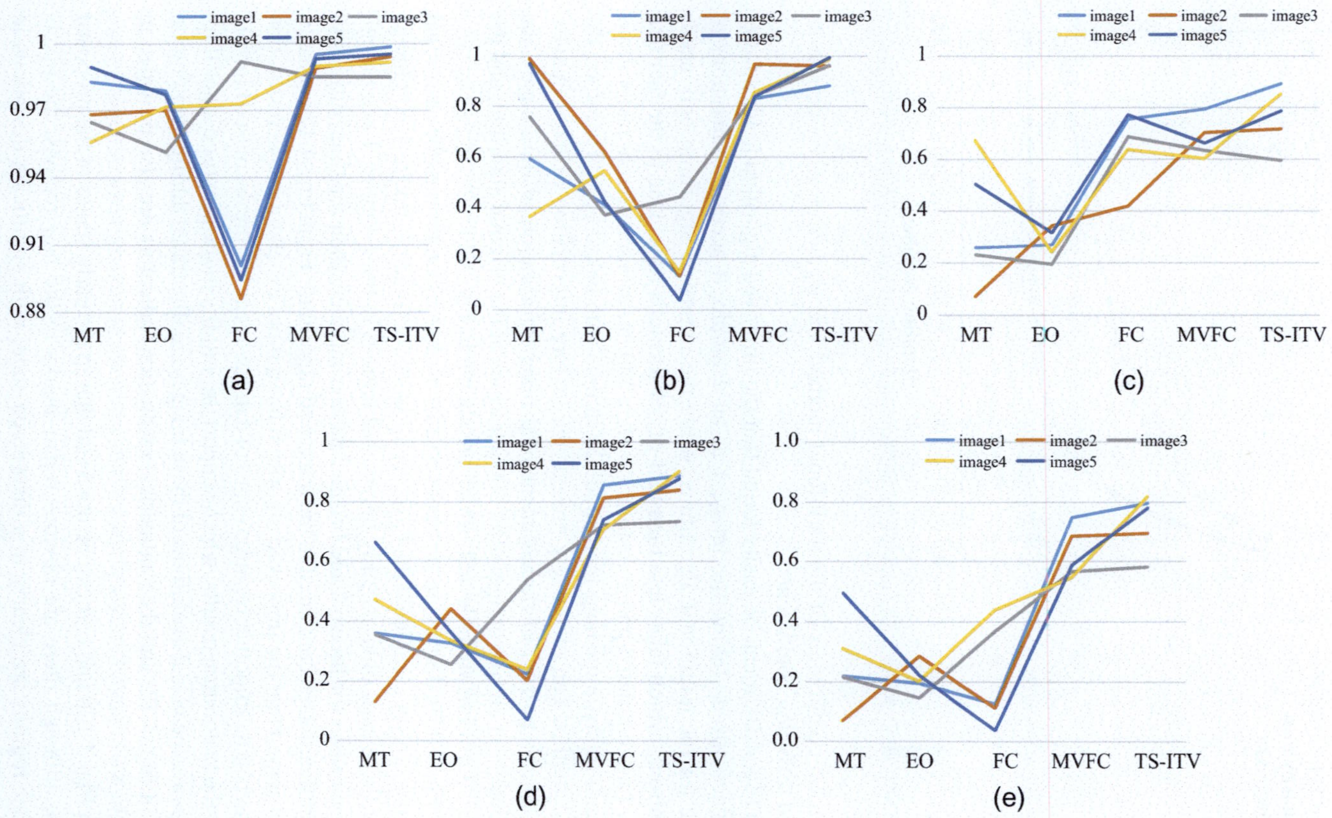


**Fig. 4.9** Evaluation indicators of experimental results (**a** pixel accuracy, **b** precision, **c** recall, **d** F1 value, **e** MIoU)

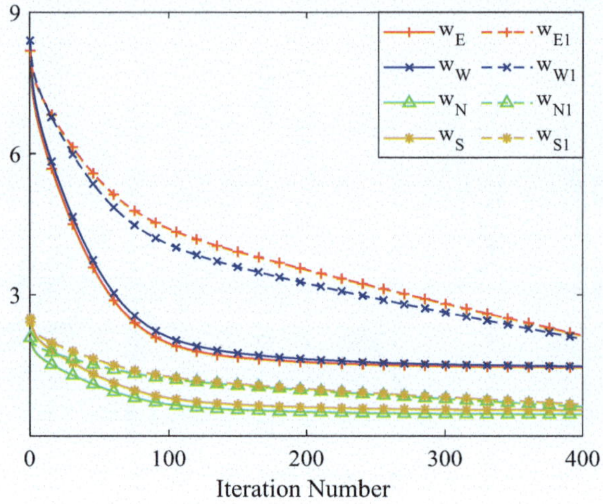


**Fig. 4.10** Convergence curves of diffusion coefficients before and after optimization by total variation method

the diffusion coefficients of the traditional method and $w_E, w_N, w_W, w_S$ denote its improved diffusion coefficients.

From Fig. 4.10, it can be easily found that the improved algorithm holds a faster convergence speed. Taking the Image 1 as an example, it needs 500 iterations to converge for the traditional algorithms, while the improved algorithm only needs 200 iterations, which takes less than half of the former's time. Due to the fact that the latter has completed image restoration after 200 iterations, different restorations are difficult in distinguishing their small deviations with naked eyes. Therefore, the proposed method can effectively present the texture information of local images. By capturing a portion of three-dimensional pixel information of the images, the texture details of all five images after 200 iterations of the original algorithm and the improved algorithm are reflected, which are shown in Fig. 4.11.

From Fig. 4.11b, d, and e, it can be observed that after 200 iterations, the traditional method has not yet completed the basic repair work for Image 1, Image 4, and Image 5, where there exist obvious gully unrepaired regions in these figures. Even though basic repair tasks for Image 2 and Image 3 have completed, their repair qualities still have significant gaps compared to the improved algorithm. From Fig. 4.12a and c, it can be observed that the improved algorithm has a more excellent image restoration effects such as its smoother repaired edges of damaged regions, the decreased blurring effect of the restoration results, which support the validity of the proposed algorithm. Furthermore, the visual evolutions of these images are illustrated during the iteration process in Fig. 4.12, and their numerical evaluation indicators are also provided in Fig. 4.13.

From Fig. 4.12b and c, it can be observed that in the early stages of the proposed iteration, although there are obvious repair marks in the hair regions, the pixels in the hair regions are clearly in a disordered state, with significant deviations in color and texture compared to the surrounding regions. As the iteration further runs,

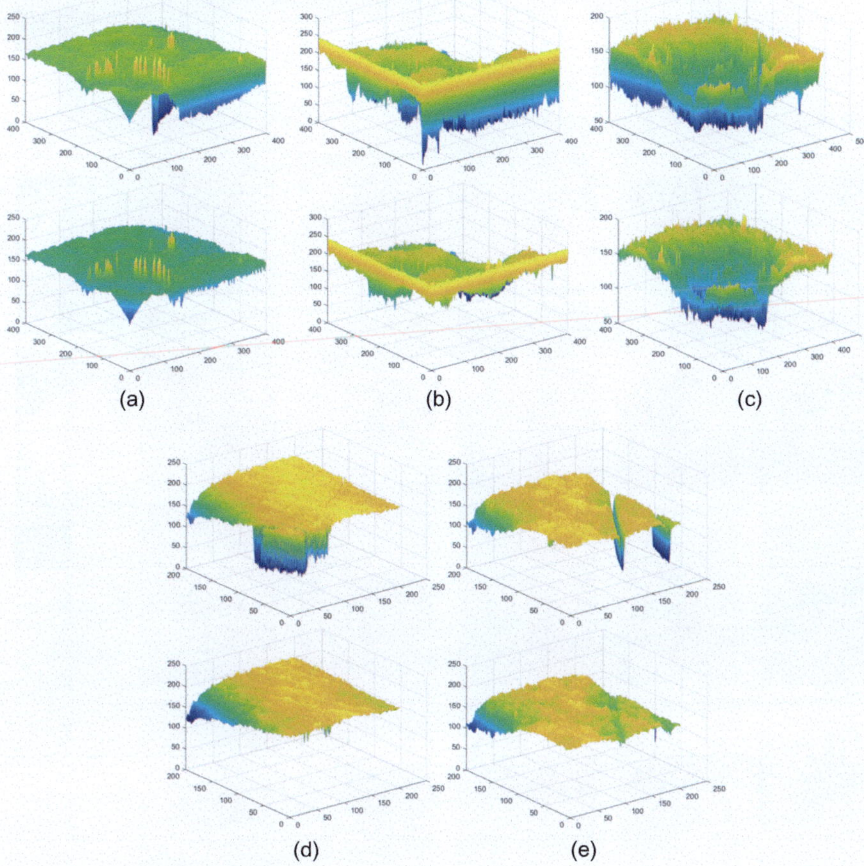


**Fig. 4.11** Detail texture displays of restoration results (**a** image 1, **b** image 2, **c** image 3, **d** image 4, **e** image 5)

the corresponding hair regions in the image are gradually repaired. After about 50 iterations, it is evident that some regions with simpler textures have been repaired, but the repaired regions are unsatisfactory in complex textures. Especially for skin lesions, there exist still obvious hair traces. After 100 iterations, it can be observed that the repaired hair region has been further improved. Except for the complex texture of Image 3, most hair regions in other 4 images have been fully repaired, which do not include the skin lesion regions. After about 200 iterations, all hair regions have been well repaired with the colors and the textures. The numerical evaluation indicators for each image are provided during the iteration process in Fig. 4.13. In the initial stage of restoration, the average gradient, the spatial frequencies, and edge intensity values of the image decrease rapidly in the first 50 iterations, and afterwards, its progress is slowly. The SNR and PSNR values begin to slowly vary only after 100 iterations. These indicate that an extremely fast iterative repair stage

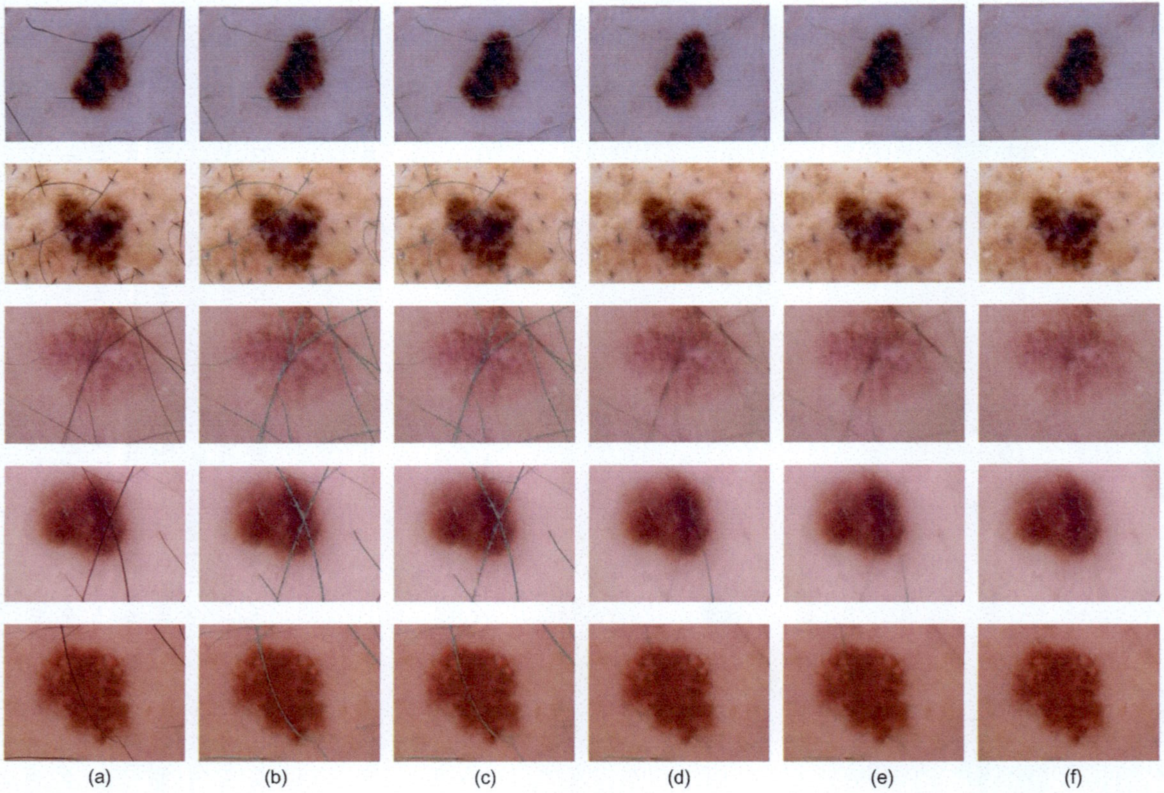


**Fig. 4.12** Iterative dermoscopic image inpainting experiment based on optimized total variation method (**a** original image, **b** 5 iterations, **c** 10 iterations, **d** 50 iterations, **e** 100 iterations, **f** 200 iterations)

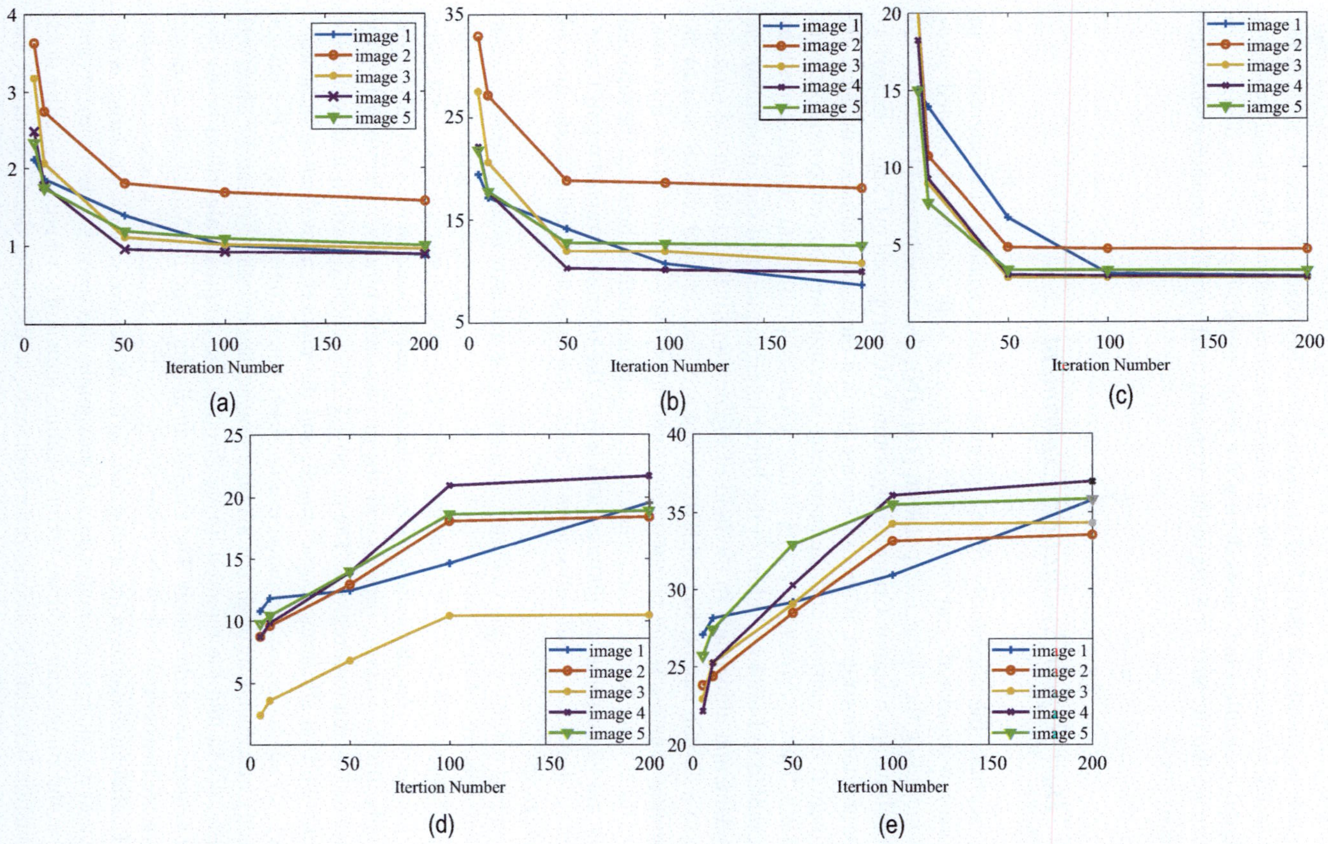


**Fig. 4.13** Evaluation index of experimental results (**a** mean gradient, **b** edge intensity, **c** spatial frequency, **d** SNR, **e** PSNR)

is carried out in the initial iteration of the image, but the repair task is not completely completed. The noisy regions of the image are still in a slow progress, and the basic repair task is completed until 100 iterations later. However, the details such as the colors and the textures are still in the process of further restore. The visual evolution and digital evaluation indicators during the image iteration process are designed to demonstrate the iterative process of the proposed total variation method and further its effectiveness.

### *4.3.3 Hair Repair Evaluation Experiment*

In this section, the superiority of the proposed total variation (TV) algorithm in hair repair is validated, and meanwhile compared with commonly existed algorithms including the linear interpolation [10] (IN), the convolution [11] (CO), and the ant colony optimization Criminisi algorithm (AC) proposed in Chap. 3, its performances are demonstrated. It needs to point out that the used evaluation metrics, the experimental data settings and the parameter selection methods are consistent with Sect. 3.3.3. The experimental results of hair repair using different existed algorithms are presented in Fig. 4.4. Although the linear interpolation and the convolution, as the fundamental algorithms in the field of repair, can fill the pixels in the repaired region to a certain extent, and achieve the color of the repaired regions near to the surrounding regions, it can be surveyed from Fig. 4.14a1–a5 and b1–b5 that none releases the texture repair, which leads to significant deviations between the repaired regions and its surrounding textures, and leaves the obvious remnant repair traces. The above drawbacks will subsequently affect the extraction and classification of lesion regions.

From Fig. 4.14c1–c5, the Criminisi algorithm, as a classic method, makes use of given information of the sample blocks to repair missing regions according to the scheduled rules, and generally completes the relational texture repair task. But there still exists some color deviations in the repaired image, because the Criminisi algorithm only fills the missing regions with the given sample blocks, rather than directly operates on the relevant regions. The proposed restoration algorithm in this chapter performs well on all dermoscopic image, and the numerical evaluation indicators for each repair result are presented in Fig. 4.15, where the similarity of the image is directly calculated through the average grayscale deviation. It can be observed from Fig. 4.15a that the repaired image through the proposed algorithm holds the lowest average pixel deviation. The Euclidean distance and the Minkovski distance in grayscale histograms reflect the color characteristics of images, where the smaller is the Euclidean distance in the histogram, so the better does, while the larger is the Minkovski distance, so the better does. For example, the second-order moments and SSIM in the image can indicate texture feature indicators, where the smaller does the deviation between the second-order moments, so the better does, conversely the larger does the SSIM, so the better does From Fig. 4.15, it can be observed that

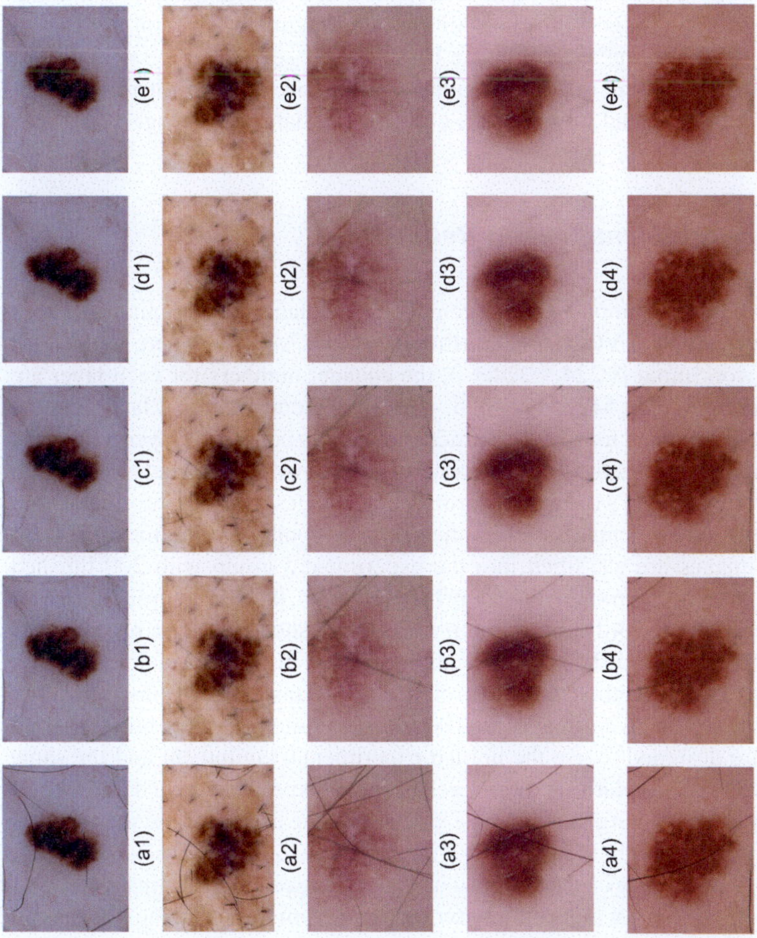


**Fig. 4.14** Dermoscopic Image hair restoration experiment results (**a** original Image, **b** IN, **c** CO, **d** AC, **e** TV, 1: image 1, 2: image 2, 3: image 3, 4: image 4, 5: image 5)

the Criminisi algorithm and the proposed total variation method both hold excellent advantages in the texture restoration, which is far superior to the interpolation and the convolution. Although the proposed total variation method is slightly better than the Criminisi algorithm, its advantage is tiny. Through contrasting between the Criminisi algorithm and the total variation algorithm, the running time is presented in repairing images in Fig. 4.16. For example, the average running time of the total variation method is 99.71 s, while the Criminisi algorithm takes more than 180 s after 200 iterations. For the same repair effects, the total variation method takes far less than the Criminisi algorithm. In addition, the maximum iteration number of the proposed total variation algorithm can be arbitrarily set, that is to say, it can be directly modified according to different image restoration accuracy, thereby further wastes the running time and improves the efficiency of data processing.

### *4.3.4 Impact on Identification Results*

In order to evaluate the impact of hair removal on melanoma recognition, a deep learning model based on VGG16 is constructed in this section, where the size of the image network input is 224 * 224 * 3, the channel numbers for each layer are respectively 64, 128, 512, 512, 512, 4096, 4096, 2, the convolutional layer and the pooling layer are designed for feature extraction, the fully connected layer is done for the classification task, all activation units are ReLu, a convolution kernel is $3 \times 3$, and a step and a fill are both 1. Two hundred dermoscopic images with hair information are designed for the experiments. Based on the proposed total variation method, these dermoscopic images are classified into the experimental group with 200 finished iterations, the 1st control group without any hair treatment, the 2nd control group with 50 finished iterations, the 3rd control group with 100 finished iterations, respectively. For verifying the impact of hair removal algorithms on the melanoma recognition, the data augmentation methods such as rotating and translating are firstly used to expand the number of given images to 1000 images before classification, and all experiments are designed to use the unified experimental equipment and the same hyperparameters such as learning rates. Each group of experiments are demanded to conduct five times for taking their average values, and the accuracy and the variance of melanoma recognition in the three experiments are recorded in Table 4.4.

From Table 4.4, it can be observed that using the proposed algorithm in this chapter and the improved Criminisi algorithm to remove hair from dermoscopic images can increase the recognition rate of melanoma about nearly 10%. The recognition rates of the 3rd control group and experimental group are the same, which are slightly higher than the 2nd control group. These indicate that under the same conditions, both algorithms synchronously improve the recognition rate of melanoma, but the improved algorithm in this chapter has a slightly higher recognition rate than the improved Criminisi algorithm after 200 iterations, but the running time is much shorter than the Criminisi algorithm. At the same time, with the requirement of slightly reducing recognition accuracy, the running time of the proposed algorithm can be reduced

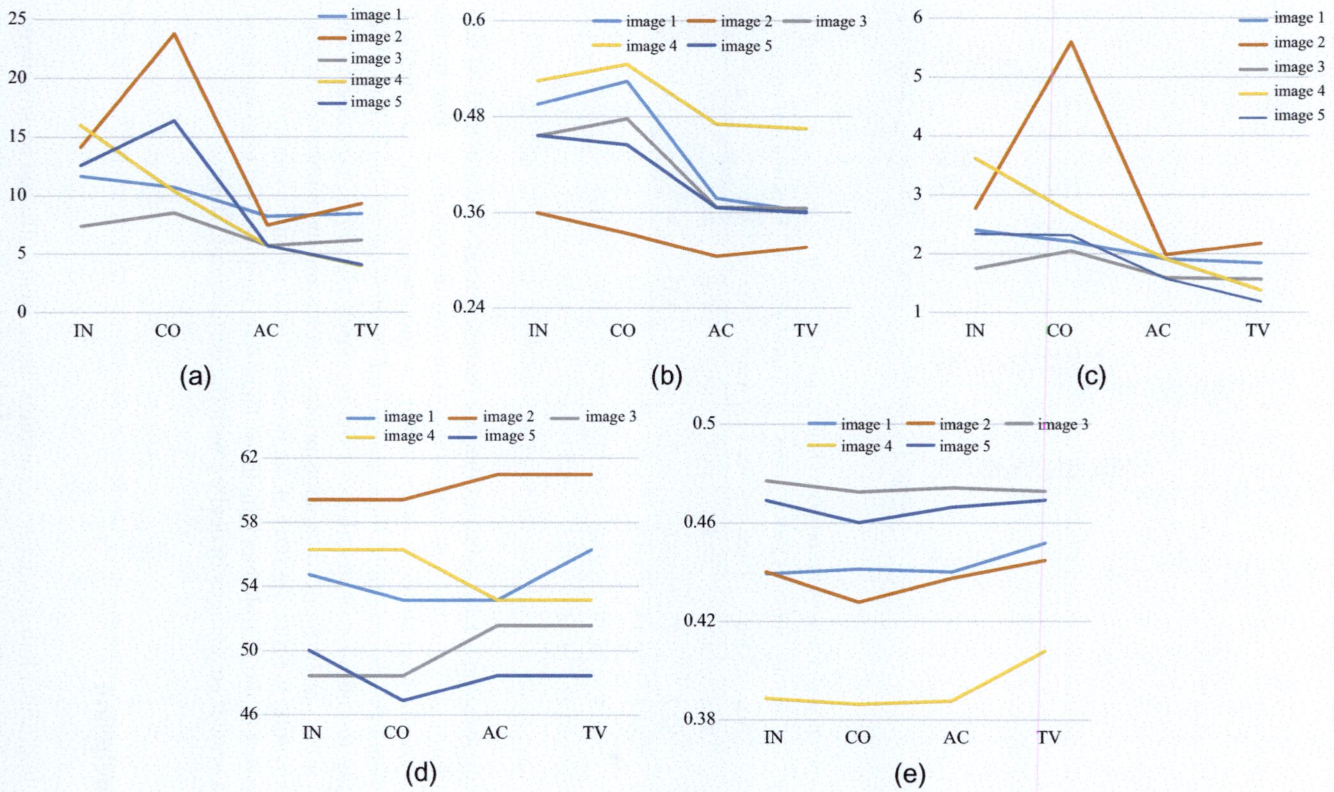


**Fig. 4.15** Evaluation index of experimental results (**a** average gray value difference, **b** gray histogram Euclidean distance, **c** color second moment difference, **d** Hamming distance, **e** structural similarity)

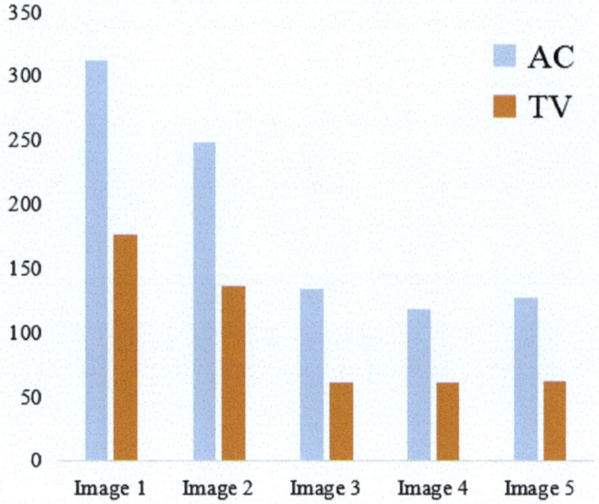


**Fig. 4.16** AC and TV algorithm running time

**Table 4.4** Experimental results of the proposed hair removal algorithm on melanoma recognition

| Group epoch | Control group 1 | | Control group 2 | | Control group 3 | | Experimental group | |
|---|---|---|---|---|---|---|---|---|
| | Acc | Var | Acc | Var | Acc | Var | Acc | Var |
| 1 | 70.4 | 4.33 | 83.8 | 1.92 | 85.2 | 4.65 | 84.7 | 4.65 |
| 5 | 82.2 | 3.27 | 88.6 | 3.97 | 89.2 | 3.11 | 89.2 | 3.11 |
| 10 | 84.6 | 2.17 | 89.2 | 1.22 | 92.2 | 3.11 | 92.2 | 3.11 |
| 20 | 86.4 | 2.28 | 93.8 | 0.55 | 91.6 | 0.89 | 91.6 | 0.89 |
| 50 | 87.2 | 1.54 | 93.5 | 0.89 | 95.2 | 1.24 | 96.1 | 1.24 |

by decreasing iterations. This indicates that the proposed total variation method has greater flexibility and is consistent with the conclusions in Sect. 4.2.2. Due to the linear narrow regions in hair repair and removal, the proposed total variation method has more advantages. For example, the required high repair accuracy can be improved by increasing the number of iterations of the proposed algorithm, conversely, the running accuracy can be reduced by appropriately decreasing the number of its iterations. Meanwhile, the running time of the proposed total variation method is much shorter than that of the sample block method. Therefore, the proposed total variation method has greater advantages in dealing with the dermoscopic images.

## 4.4 Conclusion

Due to the traditional hair extraction algorithms being easily affected by structured noise in skin lesion regions, the texture spectrum iterative tensor voting algorithm is proposed in this chapter, which combines the texture spectrum of the image with a defined attenuation function based on the angle deviation between the voter and receiver. It allows the proposed algorithm to continuously update the voting scale of the voting field during the iteration process, and thereby obtains more and more voting information of the hair structure in the dermoscopic image. For hair repairing, the prior information of hair in the dermoscopic image is firstly modeled, then an energy functional with noise constraints is established, and diffusion adjustment coefficients are designed in the regularization term. Finally, the Euler Lagrange equation is adapted to solve the proposed iterative model, and adaptive parameters that vary with the iterations are introduced to enable the algorithm to faster diffuse in the early stages of iteration, and slowly diffuses in the later stages to simultaneously improve the speed and quality of image restoration. For example, the proposed method improves the accuracy of hair extraction to about 99.28% with a certain complexity, which is much higher than other existed algorithms. The proposed restoration algorithm in this chapter are basically the same effects as the improved repair algorithm in this chapter, but its average running time is greater advantages of half time in this chapter, so it has greater advantages.

## References


1. Mahmood DAF, Mahmood HA. Artifact removal from skin dermoscopy images to support automated melanoma diagnosis. Al-Rafidain Eng J (AREJ). 2015;23(5):22–30.
2. Das P, Gangopadhyay M. Removal of hair particles from skin disease images using pixel based approach. Int J Comput Sci Inf Technol. 2015;6(5):15–6.
3. Medioni G, Lee M-S, Tang C-K. A computational framework for segmentation and grouping. Amsterdam: Elsevier; 2000.
4. Tong W-S, Tang C-K. Robust estimation of adaptive tensors of curvature by tensor voting. IEEE Trans Pattern Anal Mach Intell. 2005;27(3):434–49.
5. Eggersmann R, Stainier L, Ortiz M, et al. Model-free data-driven computational mechanics enhanced by tensor voting. Comput Methods Appl Mech Eng. 2021;373: 113499.
6. Li K, Wei Y, Yang Z, et al. Image inpainting algorithm based on TV model and evolutionary algorithm. Soft Comput. 2016;20:885–93.
7. Lee T, Ng V, Gallagher R, et al. Dullrazor®: a software approach to hair removal from images. Cancer Control Res. 1997;27(6):533–43.
8. Saugeon PS, Guillod J, Thiran JP. Towards a computer-aided diagnosis system for pigmented skin lesions. Signal Process Inst. 2003;27(1):65–78.
9. Schmid P. Segmentation of digitized dermatoscopic images by two-dimensional color clustering. Signal Process Lab Swiss Fed Inst Technol Lausanne. 1999;18(2):164–71.
10. Kiani K, Sharafat AR. E-shaver: an improved DullRazor® for digitally removing dark and light-colored hairs in dermoscopic images. Cancer Control Res. 2011;41(3):139–45.
11. Li W, Raj ANJ, Tjahjadi T, et al. Digital hair removal by deep learning for skin lesion segmentation. Pattern Recogn. 2021;117:107994.

# Chapter 5
# Registration Models

## 5.1 Introduction

Melanoma monitoring is a long-term process that involves sampling images of skin lesions at different periods to monitor changes in the appearance and distribution of lesions. Due to inevitable changes of external conditions during each sampling, the images of the same skin region collected at different time periods may also vary. For the dermatoscopy images, the position of the subject, its pose, and the lighting conditions are also difficult in matching. In addition, the body shape of specific subjects will vary over time as shown in Fig. 5.1a, and any attempt to measure the true changes of lesion appearances is more challenging. For the large size of the lesion, a single sample of dermatoscopy images is not enough, and multiple samples of the same region are required to obtain a complete lesion location, as shown in Fig. 5.1b. In order to compare the dermatoscopy images taken at different periods, it is necessary to register the images and locate the skin lesion regions in order to obtain complete skin lesion regions and achieve a standardized skin lesion detection process.

Although the SIFT [1, 2] features for image matching have been widely applied, a large number of feature descriptors are required to compare in the feature point matching stage, which causes the high computational complexity. The SURF [3] algorithm mainly accelerates the feature point detection and the descriptor computation through the integrated image methods and the fast Hessian matrix detection methods. However, how to select the determinant threshold of the Hessian matrix for the SURF algorithm and further an appropriate number of feature points is one of the key challenges in the application. In addition, the traditional feature point matching algorithms rely on the number of iterations and the set threshold in terms of accuracy. Due to the limitation of the number of iterations, the RANSAC algorithm [4] can only obtain the optimal solution at the current iteration, that is, the confidence of calculation results is positively correlated with the number of iterations. For the inconsistent views and angles in the skin lesion regions caused by multiple detecting

 
S. Guo et al., *Computer-Aided Intelligent Diagnosis of Skin Melanoma*,
https://doi.org/10.1007/978-981-96-6135-0_5

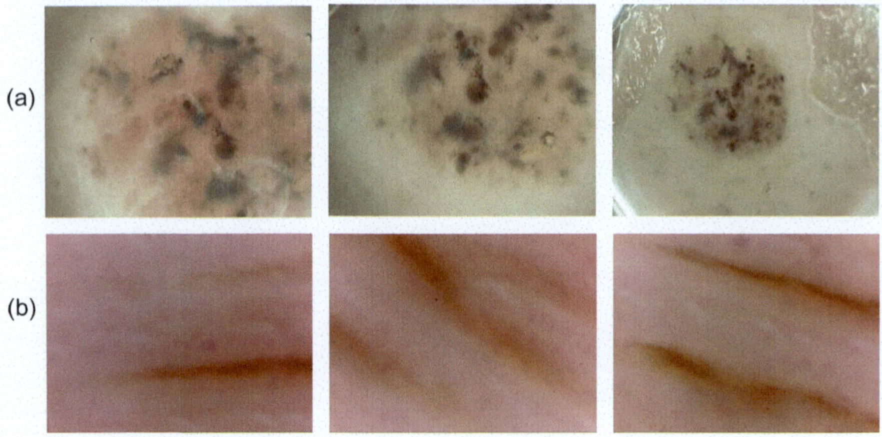


**Fig. 5.1** The existed problems in dermoscopic image registration (**a** dermoscopic images with high, medium and low resolution, **b** dermoscopic images with the same resolution and different viewing angles)

the damaged images, as well as uneven feature point extraction caused by deviations in lighting, rotation, and scale distortion, all issues affect image registration accuracy. The following focuses on the skin mirror image registration algorithm based on adaptive SURF feature extraction and weighted kernel norm minimization fusion. Firstly, the SURF algorithm is used to extract feature points from skin mirror images, and the HPO algorithm is used to adaptively calculate the number of groups and layers in the SURF algorithm, as well as the threshold of the Hessian determinant, to improve the stability and robustness of feature point extraction; Secondly, the thin plate spline model is used for image coarse registration, and an improved random sampling consistency algorithm is used to remove pseudo matching points from the feature point set obtained from coarse registration, and thereby improves the accuracy and efficiency of image registration; Finally, a weighted kernel norm fusion method is adopted to preserve the original color pixel information in the reference image and the image to be registered as much as possible, reduce the loss of the image during the stitching process, and improve the visual effect of the fused image.

## 5.2 Image Registration Fusion Model

The overall model implementation includes the following four parts: adaptive SURF feature point extraction based on HPO optimization, rough feature point matching based on thin plate spline model, pseudo matching point removal based on improved RANSAC, and fusion algorithm based on kernel norm minimization, whose overall model framework is presented in Fig. 5.2, which is a detailed introduction to its architecture and specific content as follows.

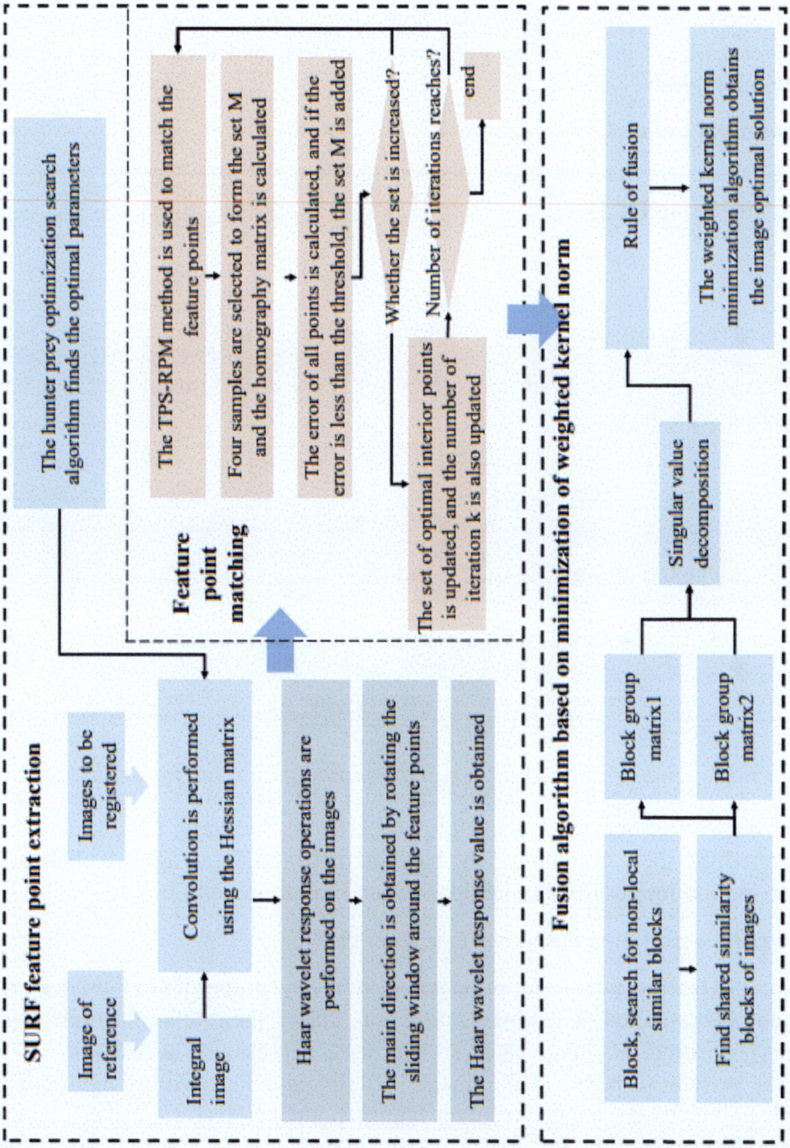


**Fig. 5.2** The dermoscopic image registration model

### 5.2.1 *Adaptive SURF Feature Point Extraction Based on HPO Optimization*

The SURF feature extraction is an improved algorithm based on SIFT, which holds a faster detection speed. The SURF feature points extraction requires firstly to detect the edge points of the image using the Hessian matrix, and then describes these obtained feature points.

- **Hessian matrix model**

The Hessian matrix is used to represent the local curvature of an image $f(x, y)$, which can be obtained using Eq. (5.1):

$$H(f(x, y)) = \begin{bmatrix} \frac{\partial^2 f}{\partial x^2} & \frac{\partial^2 f}{\partial x \partial y} \\ \frac{\partial^2 f}{\partial x \partial y} & \frac{\partial^2 f}{\partial y^2} \end{bmatrix} \tag{5.1}$$

For the discrete images, the input image $H(x, \sigma)$ is convolved through a Gaussian kernel function with the scale $\sigma$.

$$H(x, \sigma) = \begin{bmatrix} L_{xx}(x, \sigma) & L_{xy}(x, \sigma) \\ L_{xy}(x, \sigma) & L_{yy}(x, \sigma) \end{bmatrix} \tag{5.2}$$

where $L_{xx}$ is calculated through Eqs. (5.3) and (5.4).

$$L_{xx} = G(x, y, \sigma) \otimes I(x, y) \tag{5.3}$$

$$G(x, y, \sigma) = \partial^2 \frac{g(x, y, \sigma)}{\sigma x^2} \tag{5.4}$$

And $G(x, y, \sigma)$ denotes the second-order partial derivative of the Gaussian function $g(x, y, \sigma)$, and $\otimes$ denotes a convolution operation. Similarly, $L_{xy}$ and $L_{yy}$ can also be derived. Further, all points of the Hessian matrix in the image are obtained, and the corresponding positions of key points can be determined.

- Feature point description based on Haar wavelet

The main task of feature point description is to describe the properties of these feature points, and not be affected by the image direction, that is, the rotation invariance of the features is ensured. The main calculation process is presented as follows.

The Haar wavelet response of the image is firstly calculated within the regions with 6 scale unit distances located from the feature point, and its response histogram is also done. The scale of the features is calculated by Eq. (5.5):

$$s = Size_{current-Filter} \times \frac{Scale_{Base-Fliter}}{Size_{Base-Fliter}} \tag{5.5}$$

where, $s$ is the scale unit of the feature point, $Size_{current-Filter}$, $Size_{Base-Fliter}$ and $Scale_{Base-Fliter}$ respectively represent the current filtering size, the base filtering size, and the reference filtering scale.

Then, a 60° fan-shaped window with a 0.2 rad step is installed, and $dx$,$dy$ of the Haar responses of the image are overlayed to generate a vector $(m_w, \theta_w)$ as

$$m_w = \sum_w dx + \sum_w dy \tag{5.6}$$

$$\theta_w = \arctan\left(\frac{\sum_w dx}{\sum_w dy}\right) \tag{5.7}$$

When the overlayed value $m_w$ within the given window reaches to the maximum, its corresponding angle $\theta_w$ is set as the main direction. After determining the main direction of the feature points, the feature descriptor is calculated within a 20s * 20s rectangle around the given feature points.

- Adaptive optimization algorithm based on the hunter-prey parameter model

The main parameters of SURF algorithm include the number of groups, layers, and the determinant thresholds of Hessian matrix, which together determine the strength of the corresponding position features in the given image. Their different parameter combinations easily result in different numbers or intensities of extracted features. To ensure the stability of the algorithm, the hunter-prey optimizer [5] (HPO) is introduced to optimize these given parameters of the SURF algorithm based on the information of input images.

The HPO algorithm can generally be divided into the exploration process and the development process. The behavior of hunters searching and hosting for preys belongs to the exploration process, whose searching mechanism is defined as Eq. (5.8)

$$x_{i,j}(t+1) = x_{i,j}(t) + 0.5\left[\left(2CZH_{pos(j)} - x_{i,j}(t)\right) + \left(2(1-C)Z\mu(j) - x_{i,j}(t)\right)\right] \tag{5.8}$$

where, $t$ is the iteration number, $x_{i,j}(t)$ is the current position of the $i$th hunter to the $j$th prey, $x_{i,j}(t+1)$ is the next position of the $i$th hunter to the $j$th prey, Z is the adaptive adjustment parameter, $C$ is the parameter of balancing between exploration and development, and generally decreases from 1 to 0.02, $\mu_j$ is the average distance, $H_{pos(j)}$ is the position of the $j$th prey, whose relevant parameters are calculated as follows

$$\begin{aligned} P &= \vec{R}_1 < C \\ Z &= R_2 \cdot IDX + \vec{R}_3 \cdot (IDX) \\ C &= 1 - t\left(0.98/t_{\max}\right) \end{aligned} \tag{5.9}$$

where $\vec{R}_1$ and $\vec{R}_3$ are random vectors within the interval [0, 1], $t_{\max}$ is the maximum iteration number, $P$ is the index value when $\vec{R}_1 < C$, $R_2$ is a random number within [0,1], and $IDX$ is the index value of $\vec{R}_1$ that satisfies $P = 0$.

According to the general hunter-prey game rule, the farthest individual from the whole population is easily selected as a prey. However, to avoid delaying the convergence caused by repetitiously selecting preys, a novel prey location search mechanism is proposed, i.e. once the prey is captured, the total of potential prey positions soon decreases, and its next prey positions are improved by Eqs. (5.10) and (5.11).

$$k_{best} = round(C \times N);\, D_{euc(i)} = \left( \sum_{j=1}^{d} (x_{i,j} - \mu_j)^2 \right)^{\frac{1}{2}} \tag{5.10}$$

$$\vec{H}_{pos} = \vec{x}_i | i \text{ is sorted } D_{euc}(k_{best}) \tag{5.11}$$

where, $k_{best}$ is the proposed prey location search mechanism, N is the community size, $D_{euc}$ is the distance between the position of the $i$th hunter to the $j$th prey and $\mu_j$ is the $j$th prey average position.

The behaviors of preys escaping for survival belong to the development stage. Assuming that the location where the prey can safely escape is the global optimal solution, the search mechanism during the development stage is presented in Eq. (5.12).

$$x_{i,j}(t+1) = G_{best(j)} + CZ\cos(2\pi R_4) \times \left(G_{best(j)} - x_{i,j}(t)\right) \tag{5.12}$$

where, $x_{i,j}(t)$ is the current position of the $i$th hunter to the $j$th prey; $x_{i,j}(t+1)$ is the next movement position of the $i$th hunter to the $j$th prey; $G_{best(j)}$ is the global best position; $R_4$ is a random number within the interval [−1, 1].

The hunter-prey optimal updating mechanism is presented as Eq. (5.13).

$$x_{i,j}(t+1) = \begin{cases} x_{i,j}(t) + 0.5\left[\left(2CZH_{pos(j)} - x_{i,j}(t)\right) + \left(2(1-C)Z\mu(j) - x_{i,j}(t)\right)\right] & R_5 < B \\ G_{best(j)} + CZ\cos(2\pi R_4) \times \left(G_{best(j)} - x_{i,j}(t)\right) & R_5 \geq B \end{cases} \tag{5.13}$$

where, $R_5$ is a random number within the interval [0,1], and a coordination parameter $B$ is set as 0.1. When $R_5$ is less than $B$, the manager search point is considered the location of the hunter and its search mechanism is implemented. On the contrary, it is considered that the manager search point is the location of the prey, and its updating location mechanism is correspondingly carried out. In a word, the hunter-prey optimal search process is presented as Table 5.1.

**Table 5.1** Hunter-prey optimal search algorithm

| Algorithm: Hunter-prey optimal search algorithm |
|---|
| Input: the dermoscopic image images; |
| Output: the number of layers, the number of groups, the thresholds of Hessian matrix; |
| 1. To initialize the population and their locations; |
| 2. To update the balance parameter $C = 1 - t\left(0.98/t_{\max}\right)$ among the search stage and the development stage; |
| 3. Repeat |
| 4. To update the adaptive parameters; |
| 5. If $R_5 \leq B$; |
| 6. The obtained manager search point belongs to a hunter; |
| 7. $x_{i,j}(t+1) = x_{i,j}(t) + 0.5\left[\left(2CZH_{pos(j)} - x_{i,j}(t)\right) + \left(2(1-C)Z\mu(j) - x_{i,j}(t)\right)\right]$; |
| 8. Else |
| 9. The obtained manager search point belongs to a prey; |
| 10. $x_{i,j}(t+1) = G_{best(j)} + CZ\cos(2\pi R_4) \times \left(G_{best(j)} - x_{i,j}(t)\right)$; |
| 11. End if |
| 12. Until the set number of iterations or the set accuracy is reached; |
| 13. End; |

### 5.2.2 *The Dermoscopic Image Feature Point Matching*

**The feature points rough matching based on the thin plate spline model**

For the dermoscopic image registration, image stitching is mainly aimed at aligning the lesion regions collected at different angles or different times. At this time, there exists some distortions and deformations for the image to be registered relative to the reference image, rather than simply the rigid deformations. Therefore, a thin plate spline model can be used to complete the rough registration task of the feature points.

Assuming that the sets of feature points obtained from the reference images and the images to be registered are respectively $X = \{x_i | i = 1, 2, 3, \ldots, M\}$ and $Y = \{y_j | j = 1, 2, 3, \ldots, N\}$. The mapping relationship between two feature sets is expressed by a $(M+1) \times (N+1)$ matrix:

$$P = \begin{bmatrix} p_{1,1} & \cdots & p_{1,N} & p_{M,N} \\ \vdots & \ddots & \vdots & \vdots \\ p_{M,1} & \cdots & p_{M,N} & p_{M,N+1} \\ p_{M+1,1} & \cdots & p_{M+1,N} & 0 \end{bmatrix} \tag{5.14}$$

where the $M \times N$ sub-matrix in the upper left corner of the matrix $P$ represents the feature point correspondence between the reference image and the image to be registered, the last row and last column of the matrix $P$ represent whether the corresponding feature points holds singular values.

Assuming that the feature points $x_i$ of the images to be registered can be transformed into $f(x_i)$ as the feature points that matches the reference image through a designed function $f$, the minimum energy function $f^*$ and the optimal correlation matrix $P^*$ are implemented as follows:

$$\begin{aligned}\left[P^*, f^*\right] &= \arg\min E(P, f)\\ &= \arg\min\left(\sum_{j=1}^{N}\sum_{i=1}^{M} P_{ij}\left\|y_j - f(x_i)\right\|^2 + \lambda\|\Delta f\|^2\right)\end{aligned} \tag{5.15}$$

where the designed smooth constraint $\Delta f$ can be presented as

$$\|\Delta f\|^2 = \iint\left[\left(\frac{\partial^2 f}{\partial x^2}\right)^2 + 2\left(\frac{\partial^2 f}{\partial x \partial y}\right)^2 + \left(\frac{\partial^2 f}{\partial y^2}\right)^2\right]dxdy \tag{5.16}$$

and $\lambda$ is the adjustment coefficient.

The following necessary steps can be taken to solve the correlation matrix $P$:

The spatial transformation function $f(x_i)$ is firstly kept unchanged, and the corresponding point $P_{\text{ij}}$ of the left upper corner submatrix of the relevant matrix $P$ is updated as:

$$P_{ij} = \frac{1}{T}\exp\left[-\frac{\left(y_j - f(x_i)\right)^T\left(y_j - f(x_i)\right)}{2T}\right] \tag{5.17}$$

Then, the correlation matrix $P$ is kept unchanged and the spatial transformation function $f(x_i)$ is updated. At this point, the minimum energy function $f^*$ is designed as:

$$f^* = \arg\min\left(\sum_{i=1}^{M}\left\|\sum_{j=1}^{N} P_{ij}y_j - f(x_i)\right\|^2 + \lambda\|\Delta f\|^2\right) \tag{5.18}$$

The thin plate spline model can be described through determining the deformation model among the feature points by continuously repeating the above proposed steps, and the coarse registration is obtained between the reference image and the image to be registered.

- **Pseudo matching point removal based on the improved RANSAC**

Due to the distortion and the deformation of the dermoscopic images, as well as some deviations in the lesions at different times, there still exists some incorrect matching point pairs when only relying on the thin plate spline model. Therefore, the Random Sampling Consistency (RANSAC) algorithm is expected to remove the mismatched feature point pairs. It is well-known that the RANSAC algorithm relies on the iteration times and the set thresholds in terms of the model accuracy [6], which only obtains the optimal solution under the current iteration times. That is, the confidence of the obtained optimal solution is positively correlated with the designed iteration times. When the data points contain more noise or the designed model requires higher accuracy, the iteration times will exponentially increase, which will lead to spend more time on the model solution. If the iteration times are not too enough, it will easily lead to stop the iteration process before finding the optimal solution, and even result in the worse matching result.

Therefore, some important improvements have been completed towards the RANSAC algorithm, and the improved algorithm are redesigned as follows:

Step 1: The 4 data samples are randomly selected to form a set $M$ from the obtained matching points roughly registered through the thin plate spline model, where $(x, y)$ denotes the feature point position of the reference image, $(\overline{x}, \overline{y})$ denotes the feature point position of the image to be registered, and $s$ denotes the scale parameter.

The homography matrix $H = (h_{ij})_{3\times 3}$ is defined as

$$s\begin{bmatrix} \overline{x} \\ \overline{y} \\ 1 \end{bmatrix} = \begin{bmatrix} h_{11} & h_{12} & h_{13} \\ h_{21} & h_{22} & h_{23} \\ h_{31} & h_{32} & h_{33} \end{bmatrix} \begin{bmatrix} x \\ y \\ 1 \end{bmatrix} \tag{5.19}$$

Step 2: The obtained homography matrix $H$ is designed to evaluate the variances of all points in the dataset. If the variances are less than the setting threshold $\lambda$, as presented as follows

$$\sum_{i=1}^{n}\left(\overline{x}_i \frac{h_{11}x_i + h_{12}y_i + h_{13}}{h_{31}x_i + h_{32}y_i + h_{33}}\right)^2 + \left(\overline{y}_i \frac{h_{21}x_i + h_{22}y_i + h_{13}}{h_{31}x_i + h_{32}y_i + h_{33}}\right)^2 \leq \lambda \tag{5.20}$$

Then, the corresponding points need to add to the set $M$. It points out that the $n$ dimensions inter-class points follow the chi-square distribution and the thresholds $\lambda^2 = \chi_n^{-1}(\alpha)\sigma^2$ where the means are 0 and the variances are $\sigma$, and $\alpha$ denotes confidence probability.

Step 3: If the new points are added to the set $M$, the homography matrix $H$ is recalculated through returning to Step 1; otherwise, the next step needs to be considered.

Step 4: If the element number of the current interior point set is greater than the optimal interior point set, the optimal interior point set and the iteration times $k$ are respectively updated according to Eq. (5.21).

$$k = \log(1 - p)/\log(1 - w^m) \tag{5.21}$$

where, the confidence level $p$ generally ranges from 0.95 to 0.99, the ratio $m$ of interior point is generally 4, and $w$ is the minimum sample number required by the given model.

Step 5: Once the iteration times reach or exceed the given threshold $k$, the proposed algorithm ends. Otherwise, the above steps are continuously repeated until exceeding the maximum iteration threshold.

### 5.2.3 The Fusion Model Based on Weighted Kernel Norm Minimization

After completing the registration, the image to be registered is aligned with the reference based on the obtained homography matrix model, and further the above two images are concatenated together to obtain a full view image. However, due to some issues such as time delays, brightness deviation in the image acquisition process, there exist some obvious stitched marks for directly stitching the image. The existed gradual-into-gradual-out fusion algorithm can conquer these drawbacks to some extents, but only more convenient for processing left–right overlapping images. However, there exist other concatenated ways for the dermoscopic image registration except the left–right concatenation, such as the up-down concatenation, the direct internal concatenation. And simultaneously, there exist also deformations in the image stitching process, but the gradual-into-gradual-out algorithm is difficult in directly processing the image stitching. Therefore, a novel fusion algorithm with the minimum kernel norm is designed to reduce the loss of the image stitching process and improves the visual effect of the fused image. The following weighted minimum kernel norm is introduced, i.e. the block matrix $Y_j$ corresponding to the original image represented as:

$$Y_j = X_j + N_j \tag{5.22}$$

where, $X_j$ and $N_j$ represent the block matrices corresponding to the clear image and the noise image, respectively. The following solution model for the clear image can be expressed as

$$\hat{X} = \arg\min_{X} \|Y - X\|_F^2 + \|X\|_{w*} \tag{5.23}$$

where, $Y$ is a given matrix, $\|\cdot\|_F$ denotes the $F$ norm, $\|Y - X\|_F^2$ is used to measure the deviation degree between matrices $X$ and $Y$, $\|\cdot\|_{w*}$ is the weighted kernel norm, which can be expressed as:

$$\|X\|_{w,*} = \sum_i \|w_i \sigma_i(X)\|_1 \tag{5.24}$$

where, $w = [w_1, \ldots, w_m](w_i \geq 0)$ is a nonnegative weight assigned to different singular values $\sigma_i(X)$ of the matrix $X$.

With the constraints $\sigma_n(X_j) \leq \sigma_{n-1}(X_j) \leq \cdots \leq \sigma_0(X_j)$ and $0 \leq w_1 \leq \cdots \leq w_n$, the global optimal solution with the mentioned minimizing weighted kernel norm is:

$$\hat{X} = US_w(\Sigma)V^T \tag{5.25}$$

where, $\hat{X} = U\Sigma V^T$ represents the singular value decomposition of $Y$, matrices $U$, $V$ satisfy $UU^T = I$, $VV^T = I$, and $\Sigma$ is a diagonal matrix composed of singular values of matrix $Y$. The generalized soft threshold operator $S_w(\Sigma)$ with the weight vector $\omega$ and the soft threshold $w_{i,0}$ is defined as:

$$S_w(\Sigma) = \max\left(\sigma_i(X) - w_{i,0}\right) \tag{5.26}$$

In a word, many important steps for image stitching are presented as follows:

Step 1: The reference image and the image to be registered are firstly blocked, and non-local similar blocks of the source image are searched based on the block matching. Given a central pixel $r$, its region $W(r) \in R^{m\times m}$ and any region reference block $P_r \in R^{m\times m}$, the similarity of any candidate block $P_q$ can be determined through the weighted Euclidean distance $\eta_q$ as follows

$$\eta_q = \left\|P_q - P_r\right\|_{E_W} \tag{5.27}$$

For the vector $A_M = (a_i)$, the weighted Euclidean distance $\|A_M\|_{E_W} = \sqrt{\sum_{j=1}^{J} (a_j)^2/s^2}$ is defined and $s$ represents the standard deviation of $A_M$. The most similar blocks $L_W$ of $P_r$ is selected through descending $\eta_q$, which is represented as $L_W(r) = \left\{P_{q1}, P_{q2}, \ldots, P_{qk}\right\}$.

Step 2: These obtained similar blocks are stacked into a vector group, and the above operation is performed on each reference block to form a block group matrix. The block group matrices of the reference image and the image to be registered are represented as $X_1$ $X_2$.

Step 3: The shared similar block $L_W^S(r)$ is a fused adaptive region of two images $X_1X_2$, which is defined as:

$$L_W^S(r) = L_{W_1}(r) \cap L_{W_2}(r) \tag{5.28}$$

where $W_1(r)$ and $W_2(r)$ represent the same region of the different source images, respectively. Let $X_{1(r)}$ be the block group matrix constructed by similar blocks $L_W^S(r)$ belonging to $X_1$, $X_{1(r)} = U_{X_{1(r)}} \sum^{X_{1(r)}} V_{X_{1(r)}}^T$, and $X_{2(r)}$ be the block group matrix constructed by similar blocks $L_W^S(r)$ belonging to $X_2$,$X_{2(r)} = U_{X_{2(r)}} \sum^{X_{2(r)}} V_{X_{2(r)}}^T$. The constructed block group matrix $X_{F(r)}(:, i)$ represents similar blocks of $X_F$,which is defined as

$$X_{F(r)}(:, i) = \begin{cases} X_{1(r)}(:, i) & \text{if } \sum_i X_{1(r)} > \sum_i X_{2(r)} \\ w_1 X_{1(r)}(:, i) + w_2 X_{2(r)}(:, i) & \text{if } \sum_i X_{1(r)} = \sum_i X_{2(r)} \\ X_{2(r)}(:, i) & \text{if } \sum_i X_{1(r)} < \sum_i X_{2(r)} \end{cases} \tag{5.29}$$

and $i = 1, 2, \ldots, r$,$w_1$, $w_2$ are adaptive weights.

Step 4: The weighted kernel norm minimization algorithm is adapted to obtain the optimal project, and the obtained matrix is reset according to the stacked order to restore the final fused image.

## 5.3 Experiments and Analysis

### *5.3.1 Experimental Setup*

The experimental data in this chapter mainly originates from the dermatology department of the General Hospital of the People's Liberation Army of China, which includes 31 patient information with various skin diseases and more than 280 dermatoscopic images. Three sets of experiments are designed to verify the effectiveness of the improved algorithm. The first set of experiments is to verify the superiority of the algorithm in extracting image feature points. The second group of experiments is to demonstrate the rotation invariance and scale invariance of the proposed algorithm by registering the dermoscopic images from different angles. The final group of experiments is to demonstrate the effectiveness of contained information of the registered images through multi-perspective image registration.

### *5.3.2 Comparison Experiment for Feature Point Selection*

Compared with the common algorithms of image registration, the advantages of the improved feature point extraction algorithm for the dermoscopic images are verified. The results of feature point extraction by the improved algorithm are presented in several typical skin disease images in Fig. 5.3. It can be presented that the improved algorithm can uniformly extract the feature points of the dermoscopic images corresponding to different features, i.e. the total feature points are relatively stable, and about 50, and their locations contain the corner points of all images and the feature regions with prominent changes such as nevus, scar, hair and so on. And simultaneously, the distribution of feature points is relatively homogeneous, no crowded or overlapped.

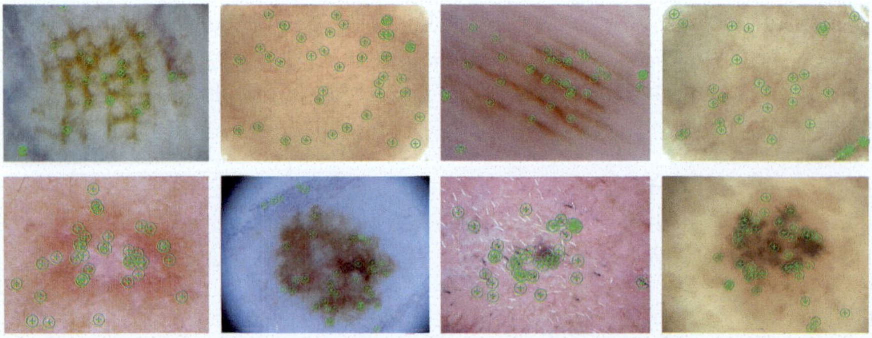

**Fig. 5.3** Feature points selection for dermoscopic images based on adaptive SURF algorithm

Furthermore, four commonly used algorithms of image registration such as Forstner, Harrisian, ORB, and BRISK algorithms are listed, where the threshold method for selecting feature points is the corresponding chosen threshold when the number of feature points in the image is close to the number of feature points in the improved algorithm. A feature point extraction experiment of the first five dermoscopic images under different common algorithms is presented in Fig. 5.4 with compared to Fig. 5.3. It can be presented the other used algorithms have a certain defect in dermoscopic feature extraction. For example, the extracted feature points are too concentrated and repetitive by the ORB algorithm, and the corner points with extremely obvious features can be only recognized, while for the remaining Forstner, Harrisian, and The BRISK algorithms, there exist obvious overlapping or uneven distributions of feature points. Even to the extent that there exists no distribution of many obvious corners or vertices in the image, which will affect the accuracy of image registration.

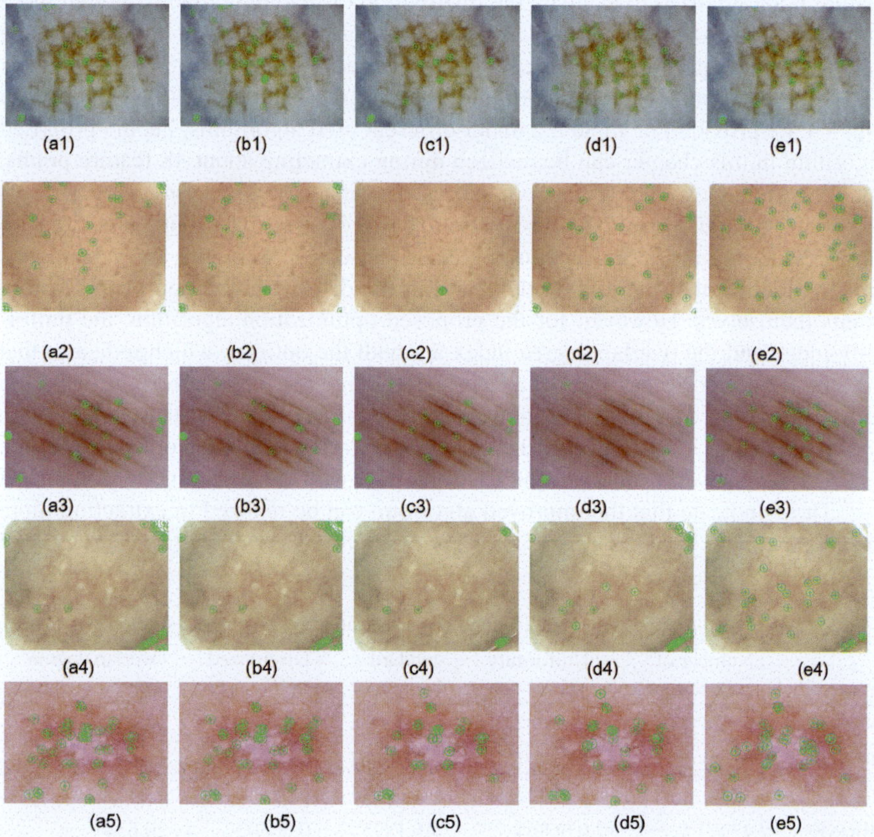


**Fig. 5.4** Compared experiments of feature point extraction in dermatoscopy images (**a** Forstner, **b** Harrian, **c** ORB, **d** BRISK, **e** ours)

Due to inability to intuitively determine the quality of feature point extraction in images, some objective indicators of these experimental results are designed to reflect the quality of feature point extraction, i.e. the uniformity index, the standard deviation, the dispersion degree, and the overlap degree of feature point distribution are mainly used to evaluate the quality of feature point extraction, where the distance among different feature points, the distance between each feature point and the nearest neighbor point, the average nearest neighbor distance of all feature points are sequentially calculated, and finally the uniformity index of the feature point set is obtained by dividing the average nearest neighbor distance among all feature points by the average distance among all points. The larger is the uniformity index, the more uniform does the distribution of feature point positions. In addition, through counting the proportion of the feature points with a less-than-5 distance to the total feature points, the overlap degree index of feature point distribution is also calculated. The smaller is the overlap degree index, the better does the feature point extraction position. By the same token, the standard deviation and the dispersion degree of feature point are tried to evaluate the distribution of feature points. Although these two indicators cannot directly evaluate the distribution of feature points, they can report the concentration of feature points to a certain extent.

The average objective evaluation indicators of the feature points obtained from Fig. 5.4 are provided in Table 5.2 under different used algorithms, i.e. the proposed algorithm in this chapter can be realized during extracting about 48 feature points, which is relatively stable in completing the image registration tasks without increasing computational complexity. From Table 5.2, it can be found that the standard deviation and the dispersion degree of these feature points are very closer, which indicates that there is no deviation in the distribution region of the feature points themselves. However, for the proposed optimization algorithm, the uniformity index and the overlap degree index are both the optimal, which indicates that the improved algorithm can be realized in extracting the most uniform distribution of feature points, and there does not basically exist any duplicate feature points. In addition, for the ORB algorithm, there exists the worst distribution uniformity index and the highest overlap degree, which is consistent with the observation by the naked eye. These indicate that the improved algorithm can be realized in extracting more excellent results.

**Table 5.2** The feature point selection evaluation for dermatoscope image registration

| | Number of feature points | Uniformity index | standard deviation | Discretized coefficient | Overlap degree (%) |
|---|---|---|---|---|---|
| Forstner | 48.2 | 0.09602 | 227.49962 | 0.58964 | 16.03 |
| Harrisian | 42.4 | 0.08694 | 235.70668 | 0.59716 | 17.616 |
| ORB | 44.4 | 0.05432 | 231.62936 | 0.68804 | 77.65 |
| BRISK | 42.8 | 0.06864 | 246.1895 | 0.60502 | 20.634 |
| Ours | 48.6 | 0.11768 | 180.03762 | 0.54322 | 8.576 |

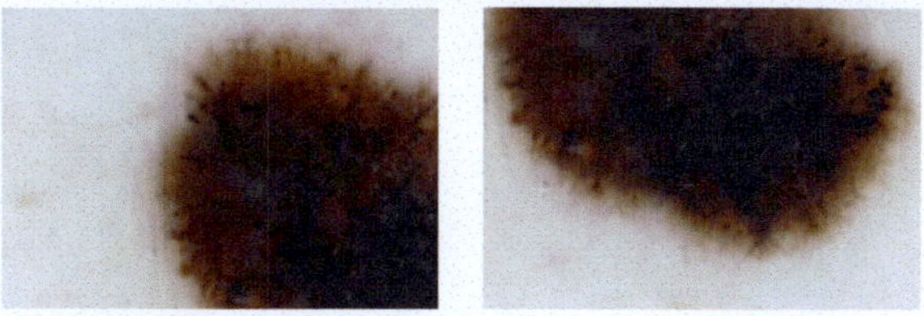

**Fig. 5.5** The original image to be registered

### 5.3.3 *Image Registration Experiments with Different Angles*

In this section, the robustness of the proposed algorithm is verified in image registration, i.e. a dermatoscope image is divided into two parts, as shown in Fig. 5.5. The left half of the image is fixed, then the right half of the image is rotated at a 30° angle per time, and the fixed left half of the image is concatenated with the rotated right half to verify the registration robustness of the image at different angles. Seven dermoscopic image registration experiments are designed at different angles in Fig. 5.6. From these seven experiments, it can be found that regardless of how much the image is rotated, the proposed optimized algorithm can stitch the image at different angles and realize to complete the image registration task well.

It is because the feature points extracted by the proposed algorithm have good invariance features, that is, the rotational invariance features. In the image registration process, they do not depend on the spatial position of the image, but only on their own feature strength and the relative positions with the other parts of the image. These can greatly improve the practicality of the proposed algorithm, and overcome the acquisition randomness of dermoscopic images at any angle or different times.

In addition to the rotation invariance, the proposed algorithm still holds the scale invariance and the affine invariance. Therefore, after scaling and various affine transformations, further five image registration experiments are provided in Fig. 5.7. Although the image to be registered has undergone scaling and affine transformations at different scales, it can be observed from Fig. 5.7b that the extracted feature points from the image are not affected by these image transformations. And simultaneously, the proposed algorithm can still accurately match the feature points to complete the image registration, which demonstrates the robustness of the proposed algorithm.

### 5.3.4 *Multi Image Registration Experiments*

Two sets of dermoscopic image registration experiments from different perspectives are provided in this section. A larger perspective reference image and three detail images to be registered at different angles are consisted for each experiment. These detail images are continuously registered with the reference image to obtain different registration results. The obtained experimental results are shown in Figs. 5.8 and

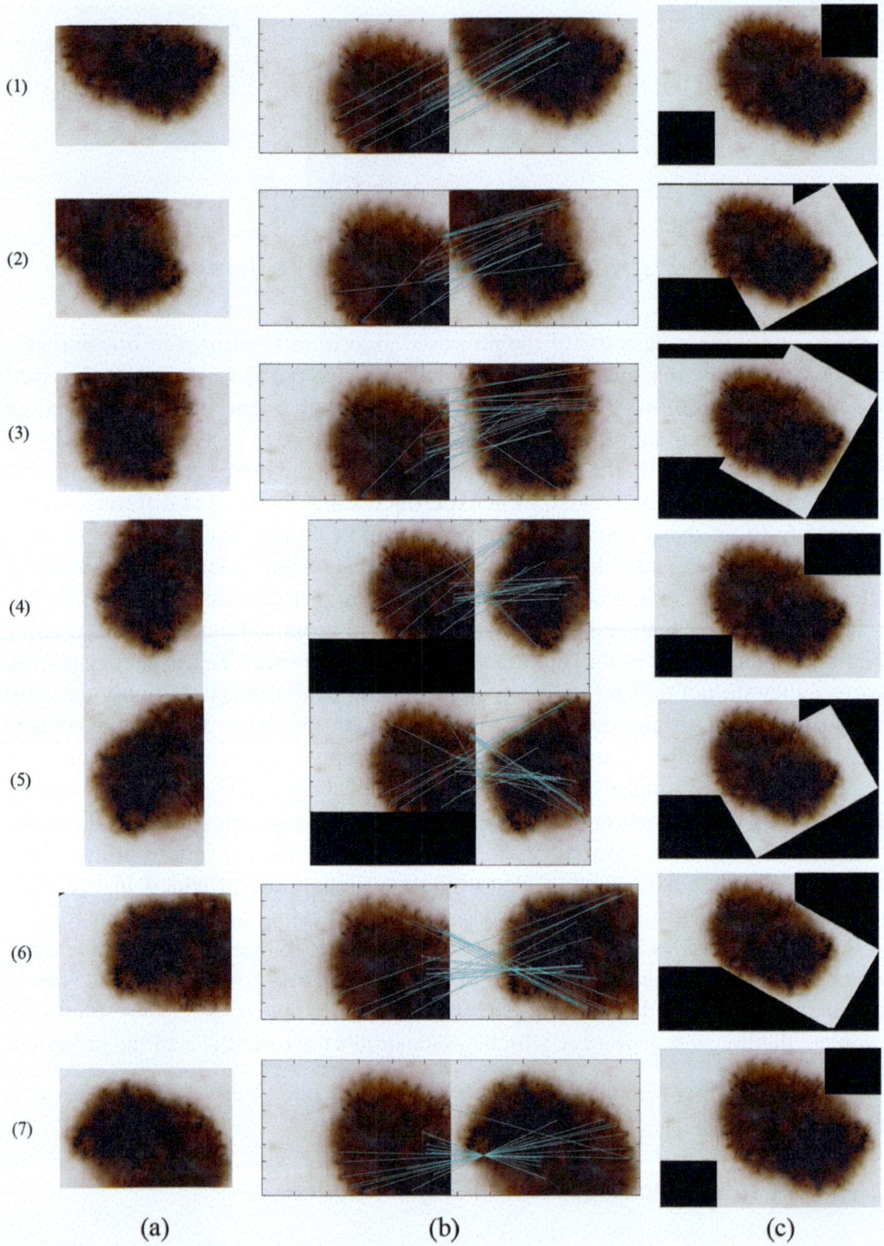


**Fig. 5.6** Seven experiments of dermoscopy image registration at different angles (**a** image to be registered, **b** registration process, **c** registration results; 1: 30°, 2: 60°, 3: 90°, 4: 120°, 5: 150°, 6: 180°, 7: 210°)

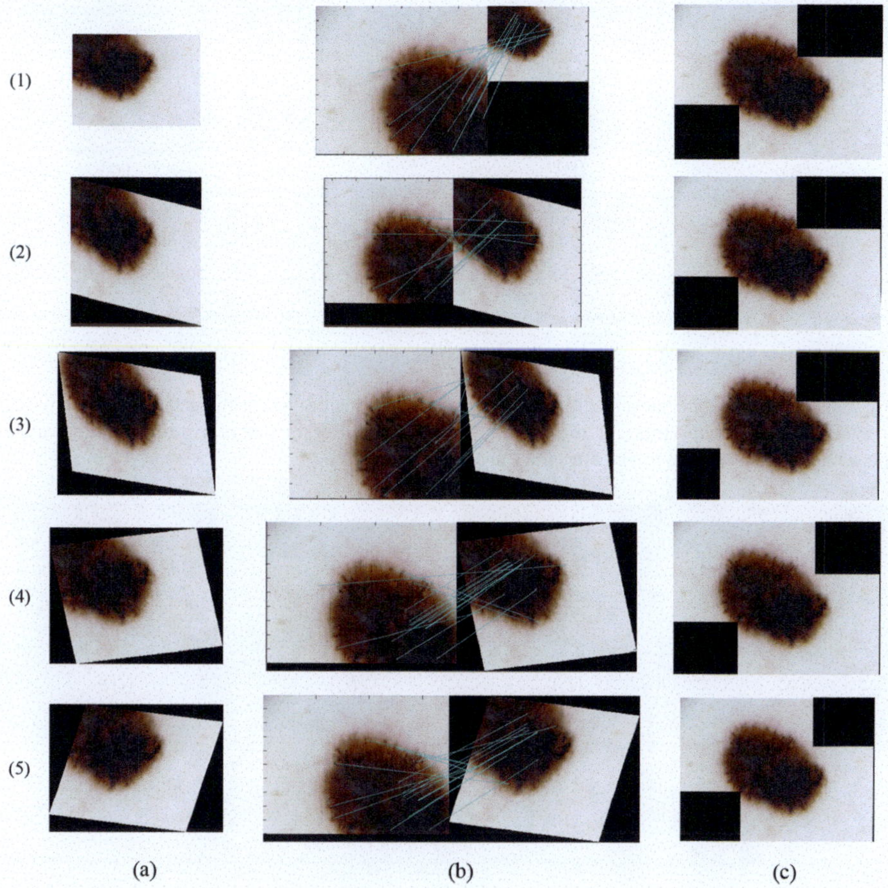


**Fig. 5.7** Experiments of dermoscopy image registration under different transformations (**a** image to be registered, **b** registration process, **c** registration results; 1: the scaling, 2–5: the affine transformation)

5.9, and the objective evaluation indicators for these experiments are provided in Tables 5.3 and 5.4 to illustrate the information improvement of the reference image after integrating the detail images. These evaluation indicators used in this section are the same as those in Sect. 2.3.2.

From Figs. 5.8 and 5.9, it can be shown that the reference image will continuously incorporated dermoscopic images with the different angle for increasing the detail information, which improves the image clearer. However, due to add limited subtle detail information, it is difficult to directly distinguish significant deviations with the naked eye. Therefore, it is necessary to further depend on the objective evaluation indicators of the image, where the average gradient, the information entropy, the edge strength, and the spatial frequency of the reference image and the registered image are provided to evaluate the improved detail information. These above indicators can

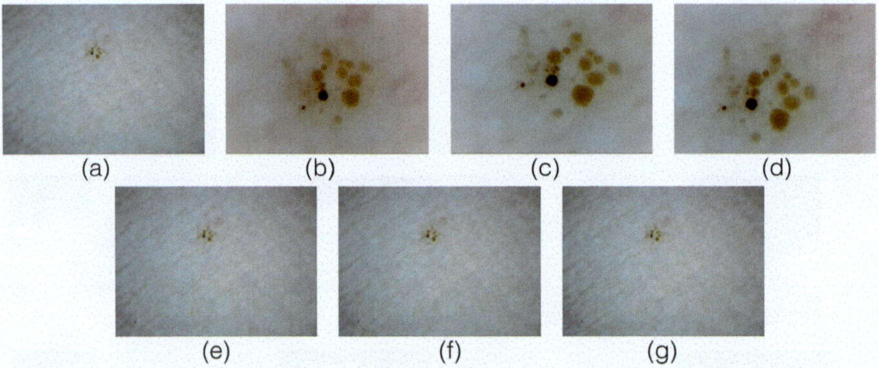


**Fig. 5.8** Multi-angle dermoscopy image registration superposition experiment 1 (**a** baseline image, **b** detail image 1, **c** detail image 2, **d** detail image 3, **e** image after the first registration, **f** image after the second registration, **g** image after the third registration)

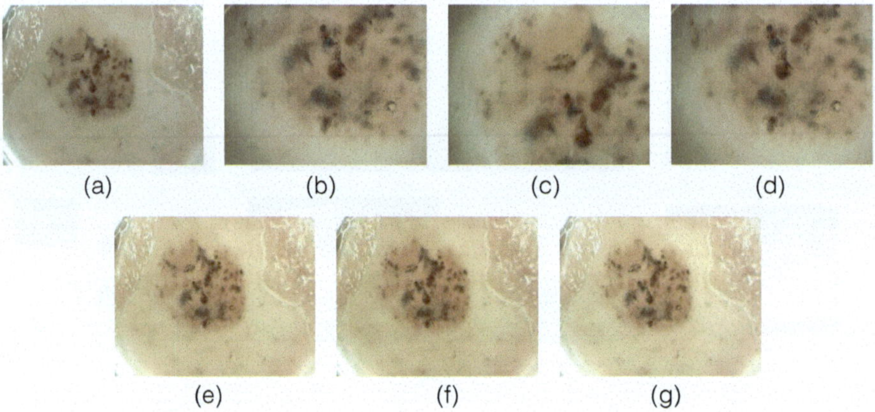


**Fig. 5.9** Multi-angle dermoscopy image registration superposition experiment 2 (**a** baseline image, **b** detail image 1, **c** detail image 2, **d** detail image 3, **e** image after the first registration, **f** image after the second registration, **g** image after the third registration)

**Table 5.3** Selection of evaluation indexes for feature points of dermoscopy image registration for Fig. 5.8

| | Average gradient | Comentropy | Edge strength | Spatial frequency |
|---|---|---|---|---|
| Reference image | 0.8483 | 5.9931 | 8.5075 | 4.6660 |
| First registration | 1.3111 | 6.0040 | 13.2720 | 4.7598 |
| Second registration | 1.7426 | 6.0067 | 17.4213 | 4.8924 |
| Third registration | 1.9666 | 6.0127 | 19.5616 | 4.9746 |

**Table 5.4** Selection of evaluation indexes for feature points of dermoscopy image registration for Fig. 5.9

| | Average gradient | Comentropy | Edge strength | Spatial frequency |
|---|---|---|---|---|
| Reference image | 1.8157 | 6.7766 | 19.1330 | 5.1475 |
| First registration | 2.5783 | 6.7828 | 26.5697 | 7.4574 |
| Second registration | 3.1367 | 6.7874 | 35.2284 | 9.7362 |
| Third registration | 3.3592 | 6.7683 | 42.9961 | 11.2140 |

illustrate the following contained detail information such as the richness, the clarity, and the edge intensity. From Table 5.4, it can be shown that the various indicators of the fused detail image have been greatly improved, and especially the maximum improvement in information happens after fusing the first image. With continuously integrating different angle detail information, the corresponding image evaluation indicators have also been further improved. But if too much details of the two mages are integrated, whose contained information is consistent, it may easily lead to the contained information of the reference image no longer increasing.

In practice, due to the fact that excessive obtained patient images, many imperfect information from different angles make the diagnosis more complex and greatly waste the storage sources of medical intelligent systems. Therefore, the detail fusion of different angle dermoscopic images can greatly improve the reference image, and further enhance the accurate diagnosis of clinician or medical intelligent systems, and greatly saves storage sources in medical information systems.

### *5.3.5 Image Registration Experiment for Multiple Skin Diseases*

Many designed registration experiments for different skin diseases are presented in this section, including abdominal basal cell carcinoma, nasal basal cell carcinoma, right hand purulent granuloma, skin junctional nevi, and heel junctional nevi. The registration effects of the proposed algorithm on dermoscopic images under different disease features are verified, whose experimental results are shown in Figs. 5.10, 5.11, 5.12, 5.13 and 5.14.

From the above simulation analysis results, it can be shown that whether the basal cell carcinoma dermoscopic image with significant skin lesion regions or the junction nevus image with less obvious skin lesion regions, the proposed optimized algorithm can effectively realize the registration task, where there are no obvious stitching marks in the concatenated regions. It means that the proposed optimized algorithm has good robust registration performance in the larger scale skin diseases, with a wider future application. Furthermore, some evaluation metrics for the accuracy of feature matching and the running time of the proposed algorithm compared to other

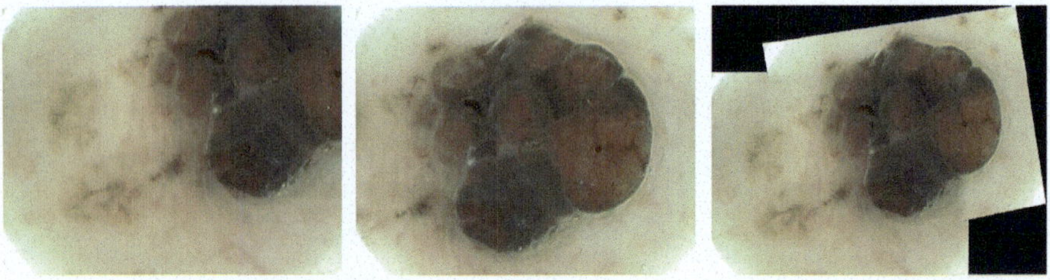

(a) (b) (c)

**Fig. 5.10** Abdominal basal cell carcinoma registration experiment (**a** reference image, **b** to be registered image, **c** registration result)

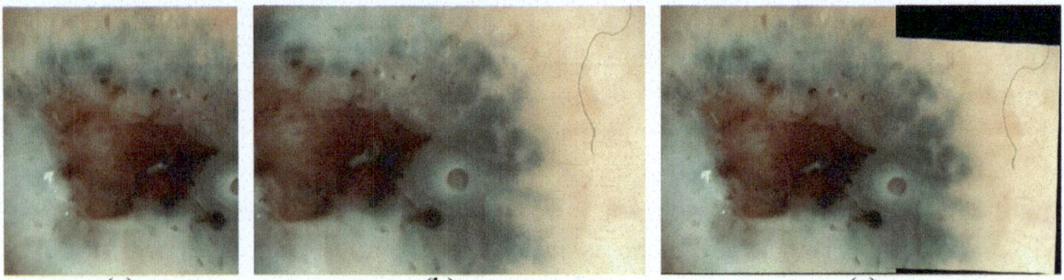

(a) (b) (c)

**Fig. 5.11** Registration experiment of nasal basal cell carcinoma (**a** reference image, **b** to be registered image, **c** registration result)

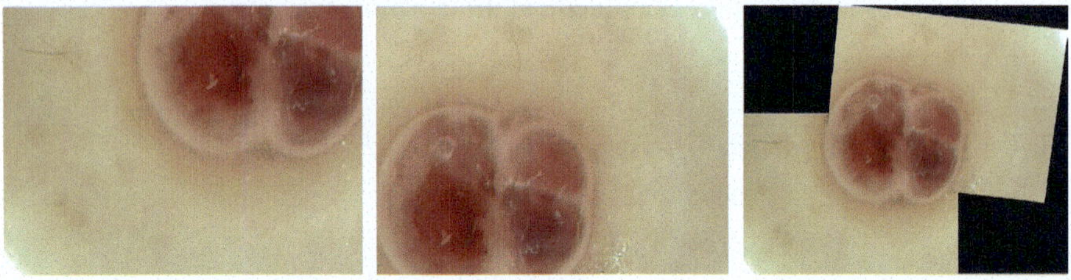

(a) (b) (c)

**Fig. 5.12** Right hand pyogenic granuloma registration experiment (**a** reference image, **b** to be registered image, **c** registration result)

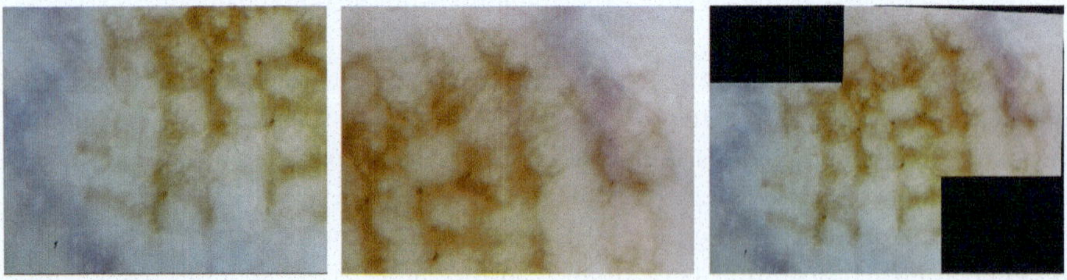

(a) (b) (c)

**Fig. 5.13** Skin junctional nevus registration experiment (**a** reference image, **b** to be registered image, **c** registration result)

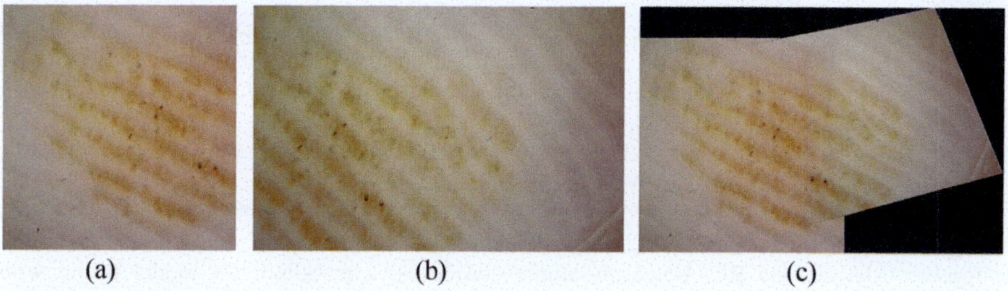

Fig. 5.14 Registration experiment of heel junction nevus (**a** reference image, **b** to be registered image, **c** registration result)

algorithms in this chapter are presented to verify the effectiveness of the improved method.

## 5.4 Conclusion

A dermoscopic image registration algorithm based on adaptive SURF feature extraction and weighted kernel norm minimization fusion is proposed in this chapter, which is tried to overcome the multi-angle dermoscopic images registration. Firstly, in order to improve the stability and robustness of feature point extraction, the SURF algorithm is proposed to extract feature points from dermoscopic images, and the hunter prey optimization algorithm is used to adaptively evaluate the number of groups, layers, and Hessian determinant thresholds in the SURF algorithm. Secondly, in order to improve the accuracy and efficiency of image registration and reduce the running time, the thin plate spline model is adapted for the coarse image registration, and at the same time, an improved random sampling consistency algorithm is used to remove pseudo matching points. And then, a weighted kernel norm fusion method is adopted to preserve the original color pixel information in the reference image and the image to be registered as much as possible, which can reduce the loss of the image and improve the visual effect of the fused image during the stitching process. Finally, the experiments are designed to show that the improved algorithms have good rotation invariance, scale invariance, and affine invariance features. The proposed algorithms can uniformly and stably extract feature points such as moles, scars, and hair. At the same time, they can apply to different interferences with good stability and robustness.

## References

1. Zhang W, Zhao Y. An improved SIFT algorithm for registration between SAR and optical images. Sci Rep. 2023;13(1):6346.

2. Ordóñez Á, Acción Á, Argüello F, et al. HSI-MSER: hyperspectral image registration algorithm based on MSER and SIFT. IEEE J Sel Top Appl Earth Observ Remote Sens. 2021;14:12061–72.
3. White RG, Perednia DA. Automatic derivation of initial match points for paired digital images of skin. Signal Process Inst. 1992;16(3):217–25.
4. Bin J, Zhang H, Bahrami Z, et al. The registration of visible and thermal images through multi-objective optimization. MOVEJ Anal. 2023;95(C):186–98.
5. Naruei I, Keynia F, Sabbagh Molahosseini A. Hunter–prey optimization: algorithm and applications. Soft Comput. 2022;26(3):1279–314.
6. Fischler MA, Bolles RC. Random sample consensus: a paradigm for model fitting with applications to image analysis and automated cartography. Commun ACM. 1981;24:381–95.

The manufacturer's authorised representative in the EU is Springer Nature Customer Service Centre GmbH, Europaplatz 3, 69115 Heidelberg, Germany. If you have any concerns regarding our products, please contact ProductSafety@springernature.com

Printed and bound by CPI Group (UK) Ltd, Croydon, CR0 4YY
01/10/2026
02225945-0008